The
EveryGirl's
Guide to Life

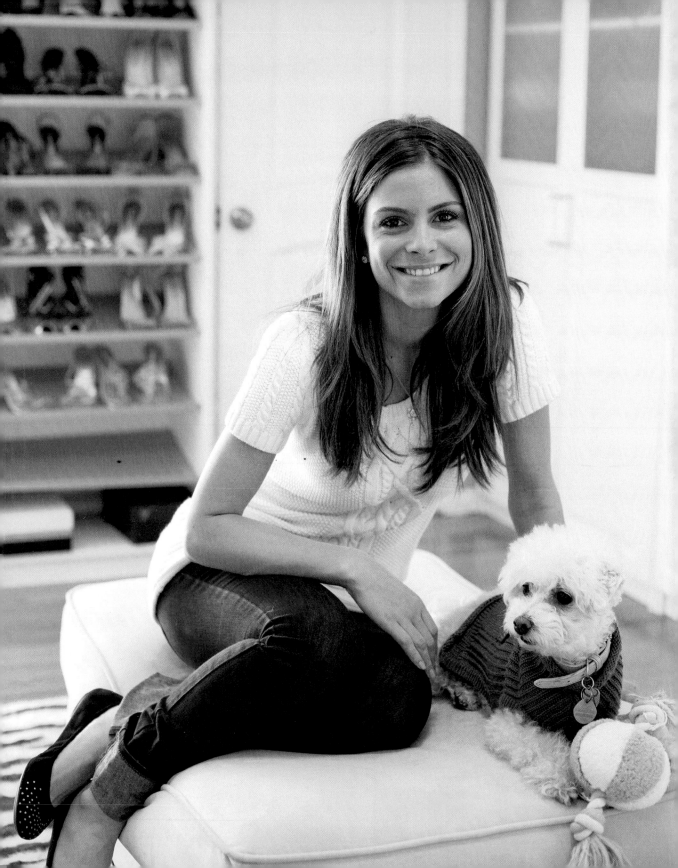

The EveryGirl's Guide to Life

MARIA MENOUNOS

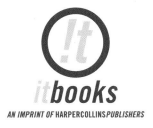

itbooks

AN IMPRINT OF HARPERCOLLINS PUBLISHERS

This book is written as a source of information only. The information contained in this book should by no means be considered a substitute for the advice, decisions, or judgment of the reader's physician or other professional adviser.

All efforts have been made to ensure the accuracy of the information contained in this book as of the date published. The author and the publisher expressly disclaim responsibility for any adverse effects arising from the use or application of the information contained herein.

HarperCollins books may be purchased for educational, business, or sales promotional use. For information please write: Special Markets Department, Harper-Collins Publishers, 10 East 53rd Street, New York, NY 10022.

FIRST EDITION

Designed by Ashley Halsey

Photos on pages vi, 64, 77, 99, 101, 105 (bottom), 119 (right), 127 © Startraksphoto.com. Photos on pages xii, 3, 28, 33 (bottom), 121 (middle), 134-136, 138, 139, 140 (top), 141, 145 (top), 149 (top), 154, 155, 156, 162, 173, 174, 215, 218 (bottom), 223, 226 (left), 235, 236-241, 244, 247, 271 (bottom), 272 © Maria Menounos. Photos on pages 146, 176-181, 184, 185 © Corey Sheehan. Photos on pages 222 (selection), 274 © Marisa Buchanan. Photos on page 222 (selection) © Andrew Scritchfield. All other photos © Elise Donoghue.

Library of Congress Cataloging-in-Publication Data is available upon request.

ISBN 978-0-06-187078-1

11 12 13 14 15   OV/RRD   10 9 8 7 6 5 4 3 2 1

To Keven
Everyone who meets you tells me
"We need to clone Keven."
I'm grateful I have the original.

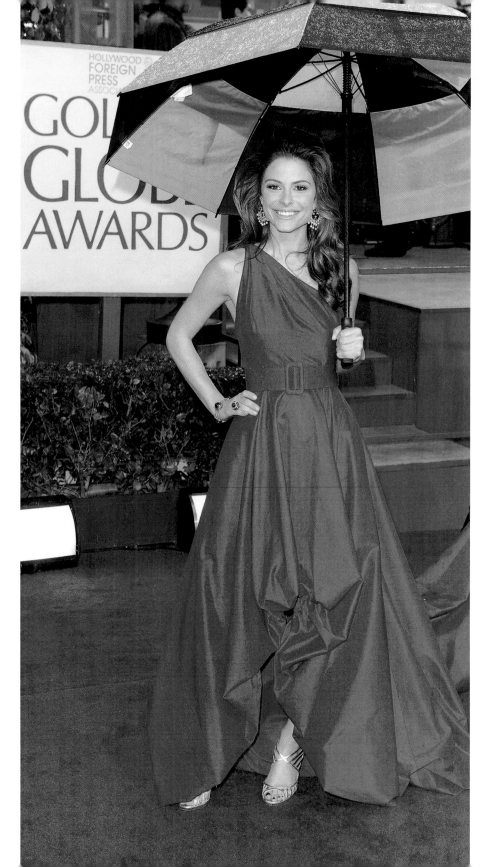

Contents

Introduction

Most of you know me from my work as a TV host, actress, spokesperson, and journalist. Whether you've caught me hosting *Entertainment Tonight*, *Access Hollywood*, or the *Today* show, or have seen me in one of your favorite flicks like *Fantastic Four*, *Kickin' It Old Skool*, or *Tropic Thunder*, or even in one of my Pantene commercials, you'll see I've been a busy girl. I realize it might be difficult to consider me an EveryGirl—especially when you see me on the red carpet with other celebrities, all done up for the cameras. But if you look at the core of my life—and that of my upbringing—you'll find that I am indeed very much like every girl, and every woman, for that matter.

Growing up, I worked as a janitor cleaning nightclubs alongside my parents, and my last job before working in Hollywood was selling sausages on the streets of Boston. These days, I eat at places like Chili's, shop at Target, work out at home (when I can), watch bad reality TV, go to bargain matinee movies, and even know my way around Home Depot. I'm not opposed to treating myself to an occasional Quarter Pounder, either. Where all other hosts have a hairstylist and a makeup artist, you may be surprised to know that, at NBC, I do my own hair and makeup. I come from a working-class background. I work long hours and am forced to wear many hats. I have a family to care for, a partner to please, and a household to manage. I have career goals. I want to be a good person, and I want to look and feel my best, too. Like most of you, I must somehow manage to do it all when there are only so many hours in the day.

And believe it or not, like most of you, I must do it all on a budget that continues to shrink with the worsening economy.

I didn't just move directly from my parents' house into a mansion in Hollywood, either. I went from my bedroom at my parents' to a dorm room to an unfinished basement I shared with multiple people to an apartment to a small fixer-upper of a house to the home I live in today, which I fixed up as well. And when it came to the fixing, I didn't have the money to hire people. I had to figure out how to do much of it myself, painting rooms in sneakers by day and interviewing celebs on the red carpet in heels by night.

In *The EveryGirl's Guide to Life*, I share experiences and practical tips that every girl, famous or not famous, wealthy or not wealthy, can apply daily toward achieving a more successful, prosperous, and healthy appearance and, most important, a more successful, prosperous, and healthy life.

I wrote this book partly because I'm constantly stopped by people at malls, at airports, and on the streets, and even by fellow celebrities. They all ask me the following questions: How did you lose forty pounds? How do you find the time to do all your various jobs? How do you stay in shape? Who dresses you? How do you always look "camera ready"? How do you deal with having to travel so much? How do you afford to live in such a nice house? These, and more, are all questions I will answer in this book.

Mainly, I wrote this book because I am continually frustrated by the sight of friends, acquaintances, and even strangers who struggle in their daily lives. They struggle to look their best, they struggle to get ahead, they struggle to manage their finances, and they struggle to manage their lives. Some turn to unhealthy habits to make themselves feel better (shopping sprees, lavish vacations, substance abuse, and bad boyfriends or partners).

I know these people so well because in many ways I was one of them. When I first moved to LA, my life was such an overwhelmed, disorganized mess that I literally ran myself into a hospital—and several times to boot. Life is hard from the get-go, and it doesn't need any help from us to make it harder, yet many of us do.

I was blessed to have immigrant parents who were hardworking, adaptive, positive, practical, frugal, and self-taught. My father began working in this country as an unskilled, non-English-speaking janitor. He maintained the firm belief that anything in life was possible, and by the time he retired, he had learned how to build an entire house, from foundation to roof. My mother, also non-English-speaking, worked alongside him on weekends and was an elementary school cafeteria worker who felt the same. By the time she retired, her school had one of the top food programs in the state thanks in part to her. Together, we micromanaged Dad's type 1 diabetes—learning about proper nutrition and developing a healthy diet rich in vegetables, which we grew in our backyard. Where most diabetics lose sight, circulation, and even limbs, Dad, in his mid-sixties, has the body of a twenty-five-year-old—six pack and all.

I've drawn heavily upon what they taught me in my journey, including their mistakes. I have wonderful mentors and friends who have positively influenced me. I'm also blessed to have a great partner in Keven Undergaro. Keven is a filmmaker whom I've been producing films and other projects with for the past twelve years. Next to my parents, he's my biggest champion. He has always believed in me, pushing and guiding me throughout my career. Many of the philosophies I go over in the book are ones I learned through him.

By landing jobs on shows like *Entertainment Tonight*, *Access Hollywood*, and *Today*, I have been exposed to Hollywood's leading experts in grooming and self-improvement, as well as some of the most successful women in the world. I've also come across bad friends and unsupportive family members who have taught me a great deal, too. From all of these people I've learned what it takes to have a more successful life and how to "do it all," accomplishing a lot on a little when time and money are in short supply.

In this book, I'll share my personal experiences, techniques, and philosophies—my own and some that have been borrowed. Since my teenage years, I've been a firm believer in learning from other people's mistakes and heeding good advice. I hope I can help the EveryGirl to be more practical, to work smarter not harder, to sacrifice now in order to succeed later, and to look better, feel better, and do better. Whether you are a successful businesswoman, a college or high school student, a housewife, someone just starting out, a retiree, or some combination of the above; whether you want to run a marathon, start a company, host a TV show, advance in your job, be a great wife or mother or both, or just feel good overall, I feel there is something in this book for you.

I firmly believe that these applied philosophies were the ones that got me here *and* they are the ones that will keep me here

The book describes how I've conducted my ever-evolving life, and I sincerely hope reading it helps you conduct yours.

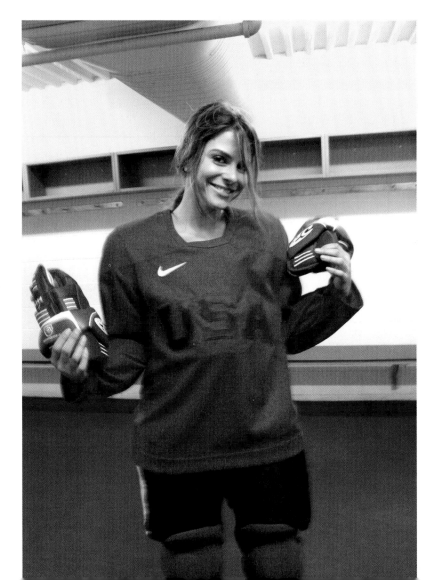

Dad always says, "You can do anything you put your mind to." Here I am at the 2010 Vancouver Olympics playing ice hockey for the first time. I scored three goals on the U.S. female goalie—or at least she "let me."

EveryGirl Mottos

Below are some EveryGirl mottos I reference in more detail throughout the book.

Learn from other's mistakes. You don't have to learn things the hard way; there are plenty of people out there who have experienced the trials and errors for you.

Maximize every resource, as well as every minute of the day, fitting in everything from fashion to family to finances to fitness.

Take a minimalist approach to such things as décor, fashion, entertainment, and travel—it's greener and cheaper, too.

Be proactive, not reactive, in life.

Carry a sense of urgency in your day.

Avoid vampires. Friends, family, or other individuals who are jealous, seek to harm you, or are just plain negative should be avoided.

Embrace "the Sunshine Committee." Friends, family, or other individuals who are positive and full of "sunshine" should be sought out and embraced.

Base decisions on worst-case scenarios; hope for the best but plan for the worst.

Run your life like a business. Your life is the corporation and you're the CEO.

Attempt to create win-win scenarios to get what you need and to get ahead.

If you're not growing, you're dying. Remain open to learning and to new experiences.

Apply kaizen, *a Japanese philosophy that focuses on continuous improvement in all aspects of life. When something in life is good or works well, remain open and challenge yourself as to how it could be improved.*

Just like savvy investing requires diversification, so do life and career. (I act, report, host, and produce in my own career.)

Set one overall goal for where you want to be in the future and try your best to have all life choices, personal or career, somehow serve this goal.

Try to act and behave as if you're at the bottom even if you're at the top.

Ask and you shall receive. Why be afraid to ask for things, when all you'll hear is a yes or a no?

In dealing with problems, personal and otherwise, always attack, do not defend. Do not defend the problem by blaming others or sitting back and accepting the consequences of it. Instead, take responsibility for your part in the problem and then attack it until you find a solution.

Apply "pattern interruption." Try applying new solutions to old problems.

Lazy people end up working the hardest. Laziness in life leads only to more work and stress.

Do the best with what you have. Getting down on yourself for stuff like not being born tall or rich is time wasted—time that could be spent truly bettering yourself.

Embrace new technology and take full advantage of the information age. Don't ge left behind.

When you're young, hang out with old people. When you're old, hang out with young people. When you're in the middle, hang out with both.

Have a diverse set of friends from all sorts of backgrounds. They will help you grow.

The closest thing to a key to happiness is organization.

And, perhaps the most important motto of all:

Minds Must Remain "in Possibility"

Serial Buddies is a movie that I produced and starred in alongside the likes of Christopher Lloyd, Artie Lange, Christopher McDonald, Kathie Lee Gifford, and a list of other greats. It's a road movie, which meant we had to shoot in lots of locations, which in turn meant lots of work; hauling trucks, costumes, props, actors, crew, and equipment through New England during alternately rainy and hot and humid days made this particular road movie even tougher to produce.

Believe it or not, the work and planning that goes into producing a feature film is the same that goes into renovating a house or putting together a wedding. All of the endeavors are tough to pull off, and no matter how much planning you do, things are always going to change or go wrong. You have to be able to roll with the punches when they do. Just imagine a better location opens up for your wedding reception or you realize that "his and hers" sinks will fit perfectly in the bathroom you're renovating—even though neither are in the original plans.

By practicing the aforementioned philosophy of *kaizen*, I review every part of a film production, from how the scenes play to how we transport equipment to what we cater for food. I am always looking for how it could all be done better. As CEO of my own corporation, the imaginary one named Maria, Inc., I try to practice this philosophy in as many areas of life as possible—filmmaking notwithstanding.

On *Serial Buddies* many of the crew were in *kaizen*. But there were some crew members who reacted negatively to suggestions for change. I had one sidebar after another with these crew members, trying to rectify the situation. It was only when venerable costar, fellow producer, actor, and minister John Comerford added what seemed like an amendment to *kaizen* that things became a bit clearer for all—including me.

John told everyone that "minds must remain *in possibility.*" At every stage, at all times, we must be open to what is possible rather than what is impossible. Long story short, one of the crew responded well and kicked it in for the last part of the shoot. The other was regrettably let go, but through the help of this philosophy, we shot an amazing film.

But this isn't *The EveryGirl's Guide to Better Filmmaking.* It's about better living. And before we embark upon our journey toward better living, we must first have our minds in the same state of possibility. When I look back at my entire life and career, I realize I've lived better and had the most success when my mind, and the minds of those around me, were in the state of possibility. Likewise, I've failed when they haven't been. Keven always said, "Why *isn't* it possible for you, Maria, to be an actress and a reporter?" Most everyone in Hollywood said it wasn't possible but Keven believed it was, and then so did I. I not only have acted in great movies and TV shows but also report for NBC *Nightly News*—the most prestigious news program in this country. Had we not had our minds in possibility, none of it would have happened.

The story behind the cover photo and design for this very book encapsulates the essence of the philosophy as well. Normally, authors and publishers spend tens of thousands of dollars hiring designers and photographers for a cover but, after reading this book, you'll know I would never follow that path. I invited my girlfriend Elise Donohue out to my house. Elise is a great photographer who took most of the photos you'll see in the book. More importantly, Elise is a positive and creative soul and a dear friend. There will be more on the value of great friends later in the book but, essentially, Elise and I talked about ideas for the cover. We came up with the idea of me standing next to the signs in one of my red carpet gowns at 11 P.M. and Elise was flying back to Boston the next afternoon.

Minds in possibility, Keven volunteered to go to Home Depot at 6 A.M. to buy fence pickets and paint for the signs while I picked out and steamed a gown from my closet. We then cut and painted the fence pickets to look like signs and attached them to one of the trees in our front yard. I did my own hair and makeup while Elise prepped her cameras for the shot. By ten o'clock we were shooting and by noon we were done. There was no art director. No set builder. No lighting person. No makeup person. No hair person. No caterer. No assistants. It was just a few friends who had fun and who had their minds in the state of possibility.

We must be open to what is possible in every area of our lives. Maybe it *is* possible to do all the things you want and need to do with limited time and money. Maybe it *is* possible to change old habits. Maybe it *is* possible to learn new ways of doing things. Maybe it *is* possible to just live better, period. And maybe there are people out there who have experienced all the shortcomings and hardships for us. Maybe they have come up with many of the solutions we need. Maybe we just need to seek those people out, as I have and continue to try to. And maybe—and this could be the hardest part of it all—maybe we need to just be open to listening to them.

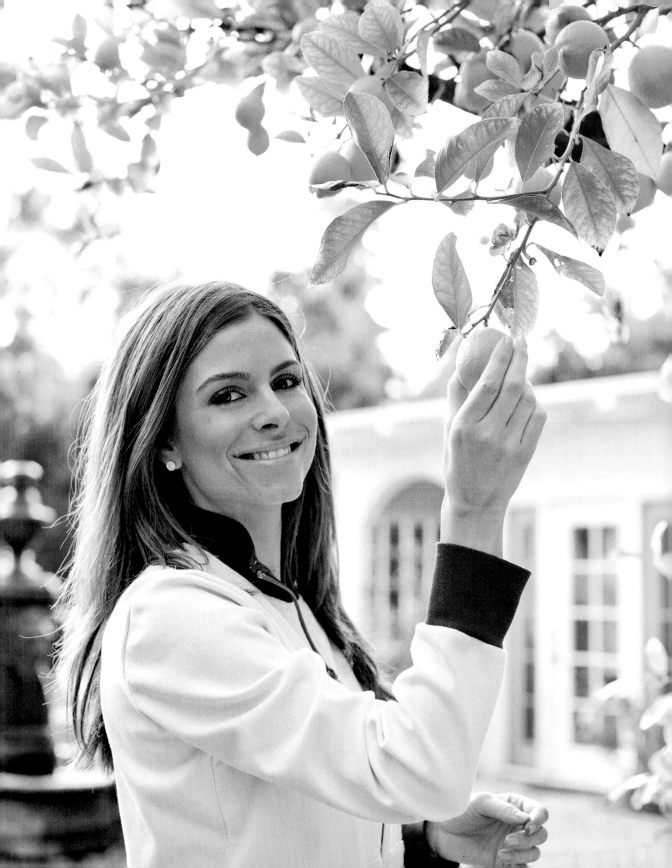

part one

The EveryGirl
Foundation

On the emotional plane, a strong foundation consists of healthy self-esteem and healthy relationships with family, partners, and friends. When you don't have those elements in place, your house is built on sand and your life has a weak foundation. I'll go into this more later on in the book, but the life foundation I refer to right now is the one on a more physical plane.

Part of this foundation is actually your house—where you live and spend up to one third of each day. Whether you have your own mansion, apartment, condo, or bedroom or live in your parents' basement, there are ways to set up your space and manage it so your foundation becomes strong.

Your House Is Not a Giant Closet

Many people treat their houses as giant closets, hampers, or in extreme cases, garbage cans. Bedrooms littered with clothes, desks covered with papers, bathroom counters scattered with products, and closets stuffed with everything you've owned since junior high school are all humongous roadblocks! Our homes are supposed to be our sanctuaries from the woes of the world. When you think of a sanctuary, do you really think of garbage and clutter?

The physical foundation of my childhood home was less than stellar. The house was always clean, but we were not organized. During tax time, it was always a struggle to find necessary bills and important receipts. If we needed tools for a job, we could never seem to find them, either. Tired and beaten down from our days of labor, being in a house that was disorganized did little to relieve our stress. The fact that the men of the house left dishes, garbage, and dirty clothes wherever they pleased only made matters much worse. Had we just taken the time to properly organize the house and to initiate routines, our lives would have been easier and more productive.

Today, Mom's house is organized and her foundation is strong. It is gratifying to me especially since I helped and advised her on how to do it with all my newfound knowledge. Her life has become simpler and more manageable even though she has a much larger house now than the one I grew up in.

Mom and me on the red carpet in Hollywood.
I styled and did both our hair and makeup!

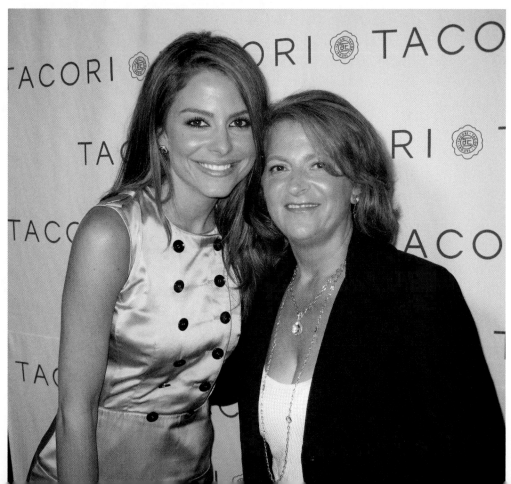

CHAPTER ONE

EveryGirl Gets Organized

My LA Story: Just Spinning My Wheels

When I first moved to LA, I thought it was faster to throw my clothes on the floor when undressing, toss mail and papers onto any and all available tabletops, and leave dishes in the sink forever—along with old food in the fridge. It was really me being lazy, but what I didn't know then is that lazy people are the ones who work the hardest in the end. I spent hours rushing around trying to find things and was always running late as a result.

I was far less productive at work than I could have been, and even worse, the way I was living was destructive. In less than a year, I'd been hospitalized four times due to a variety of symptoms that stemmed from poor nutrition and from the exhaustion of chasing my tail. I couldn't manage the workload and, as a result, I couldn't manage to eat well.

Working in the news is a tough business that involves many hours, but other successful women were able to do their jobs and not get sick. What caused me to flounder? Well, always rushing and struggling to locate clothes, keys, and files didn't help. Nor did having a sink full of dishes during those times when I wanted to cook and eat a decent meal. I was not only stressed and uncomfortable at home but I was also losing time in my day just spinning my wheels. That precious time could have been spent catching up on work or, God forbid, napping or relaxing—things successful women get to do.

The Key to Happiness

One day my friend Randal Malone asked me rhetorically if I knew the real key to happiness. Randal has had a well-traveled life. Born into a wealthy Kentucky family, he was close friends with Hollywood legends ranging from Lucille Ball to Ginger Rogers. He is a unique individual and a lot older than me—two things we should all seek in friends, but again, more on that later. Needless to say, I was a little taken aback when this well-traveled man said the key to happiness wasn't money, fame, or even health. He concluded, through his many trials and journeys, that the key to happiness is organization. Since I've become more organized, I am so much happier. Plus, with our weakening economy, we are all being forced to do more with less. The best way to achieve this is through being organized.

Now, are you ready for the best news of all? You don't need a high IQ, a college diploma, good looks, or parents with money to be organized. Being organized is just a matter of putting in some extra time and effort, which, again, saves you time and effort in the long run. People don't think it's easy, but it is, and I'll show you how.

EveryGirl Motto:
Disorganization inhibits happiness and increases stress and chances for failure.

Warning: Clutter Ahead

In my house is there junk I struggle to part with? Are there moments where my schedule is so insane that some stuff piles up? Are there times that I'm just too plain exhausted to do anything more? Yes, but I try to keep only what I need, and I make sure to set aside time the first chance I get to put stuff away. Dishes left in the sink, clothing thrown onto the floor, newspapers and magazines placed in piles, toiletries scattered about, mementos and even too many decorations and unnecessary furniture lying about are all what I consider clutter. Clutter can be worse than bathroom scum, furniture dust, and carpet mold. We need to rid ourselves of that stuff, too, but only after we have rid ourselves of clutter.

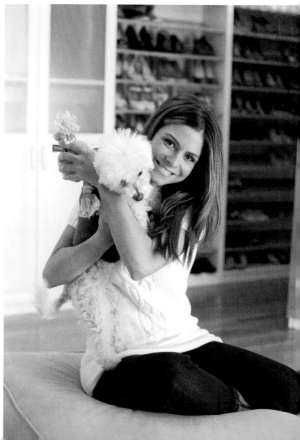

I have friends who will tell me they're depressed, and when I see their homes filled with clutter, I tell them, "Who wouldn't be depressed?" Clutter may not be the direct culprit in all cases, but it's for sure not doing anything to help. FYI, if you are someone who is in one of the above-described scenarios or even a girl who just experiences tremendous heartache, listen to your new girlfriend Maria. Decluttering and organizing your life are among the healthiest forms of medicine in coping with emotional pain.

A Maria Moment

Just last week I was cooking vegan food in my kitchen with Alicia Silverstone as part of an *Access Hollywood* segment. When we were done cooking, the producers accidentally removed all sorts of things from my counter, thinking they were items purchased for the shoot when they were mine. Gone were the spice rack I never used and a few other irrelevant items. The kitchen looked so much better without them, so I got rid of them. *By the way, Alicia, the cheesy, oozy guacamole dish was delish.*

Plan a Full-Scale Attack

So, hopefully, it's settled. The clutter has to go, and your physical foundation needs to get organized. Prepare to give up a few nights, weekends, or even vacation time. This is a full-scale attack. You'll be decluttering every part of your house, which includes closets, drawers, and storage areas. If you have only a bedroom, your task is even easier. If it's a house, then take it room by room, starting with your bedroom, then your bathroom, and then whatever place or room you call your office, and so on. Since the goal is to strengthen our physical foundations, it makes sense to begin with the room where we begin and end our days, i.e., our bedrooms and bathrooms.

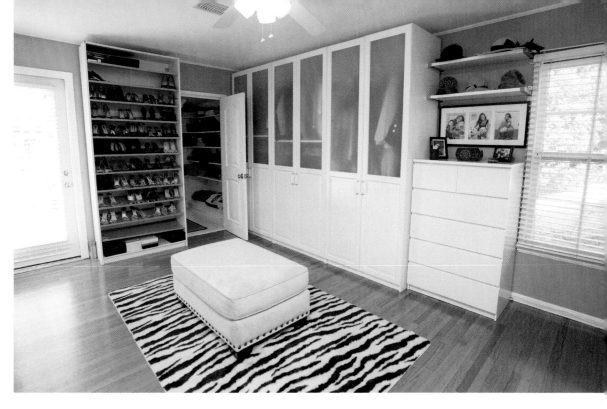

The EveryGirl Dream Closet

The big question is where will all of your clutter go? Part of the answer is transforming "clutter" into "stored items." Before clutter can become

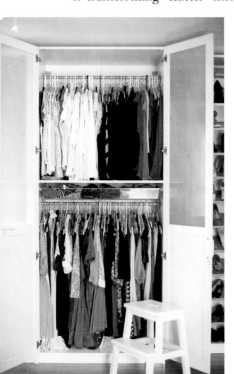

a stored item, it needs an actual place to be stored. And by stored, I don't mean stuffed away or swept under a rug or a bed. You'll need to do a full assessment of what you have for storage space, with the most attention going to your closet or closets. Is your closet set up for maximum efficiency in terms of storing what you have? So many closets could hold so much more but are designed improperly.

What you're looking for is a means to store all of your clothes and items in a way that you can see them and have access to them. If you can't see the stuff you have,

A wardrobe is to me what medical supplies are to a doctor. It's a requirement for my job. You probably don't need one this big. I built this closet using pieces from IKEA. It was way cheaper than hiring a professional and you would never know it wasn't custom-made.

EveryGirl Extra-Credit Tip: Invest time into creating a proper setup and maintenance cleaning. Believe me, I used to be a big slob. I worked hard to change and still work hard to be organized every day.

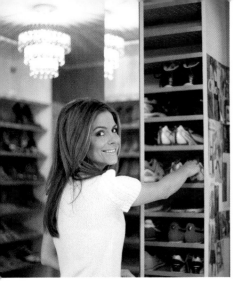

The "chandelier" is also from IKEA for less than twenty bucks

you won't use it. Worse, you may even buy something that you already have later.

Yes, you could call a closet company, but be prepared for them to charge you anywhere from a few thousand dollars up to fifteen thousand dollars. *Fifteen thousand dollars* was the actual price they quoted me. Instead, you can do it "in house" and save yourself thousands. There could be some lifting, tool use, assembly, and construction involved on your part. I know that may be scary for some of you, but it doesn't need to be. It's not hard. In fact, it's empowering to "do it yourself."

TIPS FOR CREATING THE PERFECT CLOSET

- Consider hiring someone who specializes in organization. There are many pros out there now who come to your house and completely organize all your personal effects. They'll box and file your belongings. You can find them online. It will cost you, but if you have no choice, it's money well spent.
- If you're not good at organizing, then find friends who are. If necessary, pay them each a day's wage or barter or offer to do something for them in return.
- Schedule an actual date and time to start your project. Don't put it off for "someday."
- To find different ways to organize your closet, search the Web, look through decorating magazines, and visit stores like IKEA, Lowe's, and Home Depot.
- Do you want several poles or perhaps cubes? Maybe you want a drawer system. Assess what makes sense for your lifestyle and the type of items you store in your closet.
- Organize your closet by groups, including jeans, skirts, dresses, and shoes. Color-match items within those groups. All your pink shirts will now be living together, as will all of your jeans.
- Make sure that everything in that closet has a place. There will be no more "free throws" and letting the shoes and skirts land "wherever." Expensive purses always come with purse bags. Those are their homes. Make sure your things are always returned to their homes.

The Handy EveryGirl

Sure, boyfriends, hubbies, and parents or a big fat checking account can do this kind of work for you. But what happens when one day, worst-case scenario, God forbid, there are no boyfriends, hubbies, or parents to do it for you? What if the fat bank account has suddenly grown thin?

The needier you are, the more apt you'll be to settle on partners who aren't right for you. I knew a girl who literally let her drunken and abusive husband back into her house just because she couldn't handle doing, as she put it, "the guy things around the house."

Engaging in these tasks doesn't empowers you in just personal choices; it empowers you in business ones, too. The confidence I get from being handy and from knowing I can take care of myself is a confidence that extends to my work. If I lost my job, I'd manage. I'd downgrade to another fixer-upper and would clean the house and mow the grass myself. If you need added motivation, I don't know a guy out there who doesn't admire a woman who can do things for herself.

The EveryGirl Toolbox

Tools are something you need to buy and to always have on hand. You don't need a machine shop, just a hammer, a tape measure, pliers, and a screwdriver with detachable heads. Tool kits come in plastic suitcases and are sold at Target for under forty dollars. In addition, pick up an electric or battery-operated drill, for as low as thirty dollars, and a set of drill and screw bits, for as low as ten dollars. These drills are lightweight and convenient for hanging items, in addition to completing many other projects.

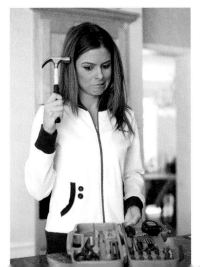
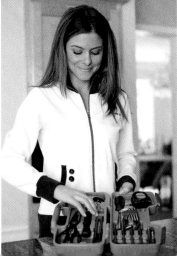
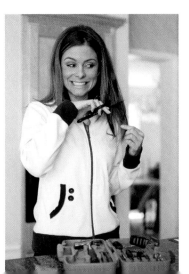

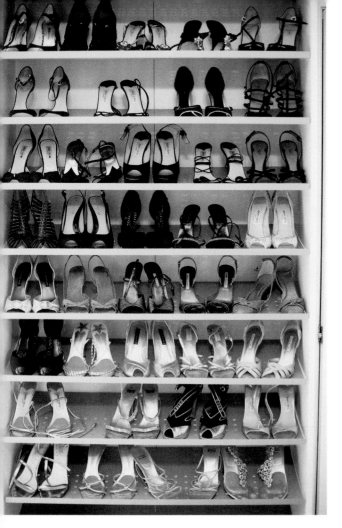

Build Your Closet

When creating your closet, sketch out what extra shelves need to be created or what extra poles need to be put in. If you are someone who can't visualize this sort of thing, then call in a friend or a friend of a friend who can. Don't be afraid to go to places like Lowe's, IKEA, or Home Depot to look at displays. They have all the clips, brackets, shelves, poles, and attachments you'll need and the tools to do it, too.

As you design your closets, remember what I made you ask yourself earlier. Is the closet designed to maximize every inch of space available? For instance, can you get a second pole in below the one you have? One place that can also be overlooked is the backs of closet doors. These are amazing spaces for hanging wire shoe racks (available at any of the above-mentioned stores) or long mirrors. If you need shelves cut to a certain size, Home Depot or Lowe's can cut them for you. By having them cut for you, the shelves are easier to transport home, too. They have white shelves in their closet section, but you can also just use finished plywood and paint it if necessary.

For installing shelves and shelf brackets, you'll probably need to pick up some plastic anchors. These anchors are just plastic sleeves that you insert into predrilled holes (holes you can easily drill with your new drill) in your wall. Once inserted, screws can be screwed into them to firmly attach the bracket that will hold your shelf. The bigger the anchor, the more weight it can hold. Anchors are also great to use when hanging heavy paintings and mirrors. I'd be lying if I said I could hang Sheetrock. Still, I can manage to drill holes and turn screws, and that's the most you'll probably need to do. Workers at Home Depot or Lowe's can usually advise you on what to do and what to buy. If the task is too daunting, then as I said, enlist a friend or parent if need be. Just get it done.

Or Just Buy One

If your bedroom closet isn't big enough, then consider the closets that you can buy, construct, and place in your room, as I have for my home. IKEA has an amazing selection. These require heavy lifting and construction, but there are companies and individuals who get paid a nominal fee to construct them. They'll do it better and faster than you, too. Look online or ask a clerk at IKEA to find one. If it seems pricey, remember it's far less than a closet company would charge, and it's something you'll be using for many years that will improve the quality of your life.

Keven and I bought everything we needed at IKEA. We assembled it all together: cabinets, mirrors, dressers, and shoe racks. We lined the perimeter of my office with the units, and added a rug and an ottoman, too. With a small amount of money and some extra space, I can get ready in a comfortable environment. I know I'm lucky to have a spare room for a dream closet, but yours can double as an office (mine did for years) or you can have a setup like this in your bedroom.

Label your jeans, for example, SKINNY *or* WIDE LEG. *I also do it by size!*

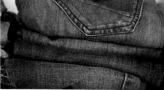

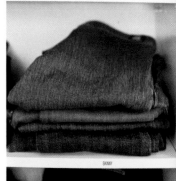

Stacked IKEA nightstands hold my jewelry, sunglasses, and other accessories. I have found that hanging purses is a great way to keep them neat.

Jewelry trays keep everything tidy.

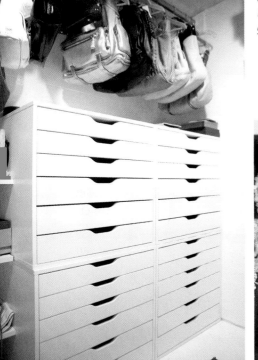

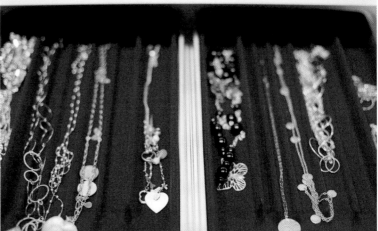

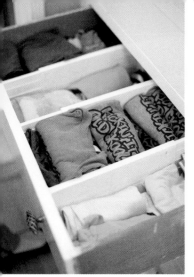

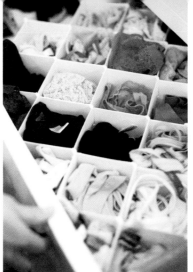

Dividers are a great way to organize T-shirts.

Drawers and Cabinets

Now that our closets are maximized to properly hold our stored items, let's do the same for drawers and cabinets. Once again, Home Depot and Lowe's have some neat items to help you, but so do Target, Bed Bath & Beyond, and the Container Store. There are great innovations out there, such as drawer dividers and cabinet organizers. The same rule applies. What we don't see we won't use, so let's make sure that when we do open cabinets and drawers, we see everything.

Accessories

I use dividers for my underwear to keep them from becoming messy in a drawer. For my belts, I bought four nightstands with thin drawers from IKEA that I keep inside my closet. I have a dresser, which I also bought at IKEA, for jewelry and sunglasses. I use jewelry trays from Lowe's to lay all the items out. Another jewelry organizer I love is the hanging jewelry bag. When I didn't have the space, the hanging jewelry bag was a lifesaver. All the jewelry was in clear view and easily accessible.

EveryGirl Extra-Credit Tip: Create little dividers between hangers, as is done in clothing stores. Have the dividers separate sizes and make corresponding notes on them: SWEATERS, BLAZERS, and so forth.

Organize Your Jeans

I keep jeans on shelves and organize them by style, labeling each shelf for skinny jeans, wide-leg jeans, jeans for flats, comfy and casual jeans and so on. No longer am I fishing through tons of jeans. This makes getting ready faster and easier. When I recently interviewed Jen Utley, wife of Philadelphia Phillies star Chase Utley and former stylist for *Access Hollywood*, I took a tour of her beautiful house. When I told her of my system, she flipped.

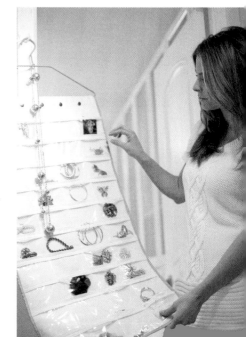

As for my other clothes, I have one rack each designated for blouses, dresses, button-downs, sweaters, sweat suits, blazers, and so forth. I have a ton of clothes because of my job, but you can still use the same system. When I was at *ET* and living in my first house, I had a small closet and dresser, but I made it work.

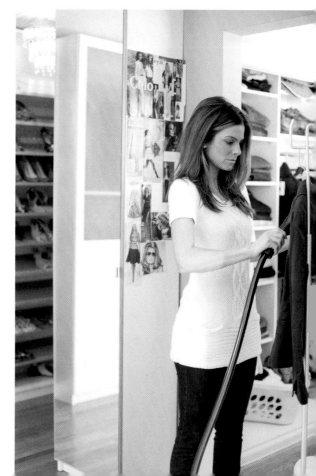

I haven't used an iron in years!

EveryGirl Gotta Have It: A Stand-up Steamer

Just like all the pro stylists, I have a stand-up steamer, which I bought at Bed Bath & Beyond. The speed, ease, and efficiency are amazing and beat ironing. I also take a travel-size one on the road with me. Or just hang the item in the bathroom when taking a steamy shower—that always does the trick in a jam.

Find Hidden Space, Create Hidden Storage

A great place for storage is under the bed. I find that long plastic boxes with flip-open lids—the kind used to store wrapping paper—make excellent storage units for this purpose. I keep three of these under my bed and easily slide them out when needed. They're ideal for things you don't use every day or for things you use while in your bedroom, such as heating pads, extra linens, or even workout gear. You can find these and other handy storage gadgets at the Container Store.

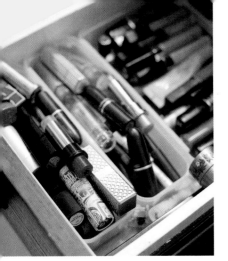

Bathroom

My makeup is organized in my bathroom drawers, and each drawer has its own dividers. Face products, like foundation, bronzers, powders, and concealers, are in one drawer; eye shadows, liners, and mascaras are in another; lipsticks, balms, lip liners in another; and all skin stuff, such as moisturizers and eye creams, are in another. I keep all my hair products in a basket inside the cabinet. Brushes and combs are in their own separate drawer. A few years ago, I won the *Spike Video Games Awards'* Cyber Vixen of the Year award. The trophy is a gold monkey holding a joystick. All of my headbands hang from the monkey's crown. It works for me!

Face Cloths and Hampers

On the counter, I have a basket for my face towels, and each towel is rolled up to give my bathroom that high-end hotel feel. I like my hamper close to where I undress.

EveryGirl Gotta Have It: A Labeler

I remember visiting Ying Chu for *Seventeen* magazine. Dynamic, pretty, and successful, Ying showed me a major part of *her* foundation—her office. I walked in, and besides noticing that it was beyond organized and beyond Zen, I saw that pretty much everything had a printed label. For example, she had these little white cardboard boxes from IKEA labeled to store a variety of useful items. She never had to worry about where things were, and the place looked so neat.

I applied her technique to my office, as well as my closets, drawers, shelves, and storage areas. This helps you and others, roommates, parents, partners, children, housekeepers, babysitters, or nannies, to put things back in their proper places.

I label so many things, and as a result, I always know where everything in my life is, as do the people who live with me and work with me. Labeling is so important that I highly recommend you purchase a labeler of some kind. A printed label will look sleeker, neater, and more professional than a handwritten label. Another useful tip—create RETURN TO labels. Stuff like staplers and calculators seem to end up in every room of the house other than the room I need them to be in, namely my office. I label many things RETURN TO MARIA'S OFFICE or RETURN TO KITCHEN or RETURN TO FAMILY ROOM.

Cleanup

Our respective storage areas are in order. The next thing we need to do is buy a box of heavy-duty trash bags, then roll up our sleeves and engage in one massive cleanup. Starting with our bedrooms, we'll separate clutter into four piles.

One pile should be designated for items to be donated to friends or charity. A second pile is for those items to be sold on places such as eBay or Craigslist. A third pile is for those items you wish to keep but need merely to store properly. A fourth pile is for trash, e.g., loose papers or broken items. In assessing your clutter and what item goes into what pile, think about wh at it is you really and truly need.

REMEMBER YOUR PILES

1. Give away
2. Sell on eBay or Craigslist
3. Store properly
4. Toss (but see 1 again, and try to give away)

"Keep anything that FITS, is in GREAT condition, and is a true modern classic. In other words, either a great basic OR something that belongs to a 'recyclable' trend: things that come back over and over again. For example, but not limited to: tweed, military, floral, black, mod, hippie, biker, punk, nautical, etc."

—Stacy London,
cohost of TLC's What Not to Wear *and cofounder of* Style For Hire

Now put everything into its proper place. Be careful to put items you use most into the most accessible areas. Items such as Christmas decorations or high school yearbooks can be stored in those harder-to-reach, harder-to-view places.

EveryGirl Extra-Credit Tip: A charitable donation will enable you to receive tax credit (so long as it's a legal 501(c)(3) charitable organization and you receive a receipt).

EveryGirl Extra-Credit Tip: There are companies out there that specialize in junk removal if your city or town isn't set up for it. Check online for them. Also call your trash-removal company, and for a low fee they will probably do a bulk pickup, which you must schedule. It's a great way to remove a lot and pay very little.

Stock Up on What You Need

When I was living paycheck to paycheck, it was hard to buy in bulk and stock up. But if you can afford it, then do it. It means fewer errands to run and less chance of reaching for something you need and not having it—which is the worst. I buy everyday staple items in bulk (lightbulbs, batteries, cleaning supplies, toiletries, etc.).

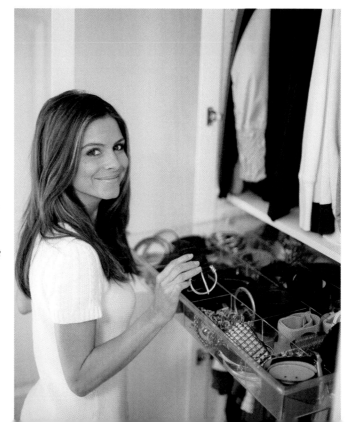

I keep all of my belts in this tray. Hanging them is a recipe for disaster. Inevitably you'll want the one in the back and leave behind a mess of belts you didn't have time to put away.

The EveryGirl Office

Whether you're a businesswoman or a mother, you must have some kind of office set up to manage your life. Hopefully, you have a separate room that can serve as your office. Bedrooms are for sleeping. Having work-related things in bedrooms, such as a desk or office setup, can strain the mind and, therefore, conflict with sleep. Still, if it's all you have available, you can make it work. When I lived with my parents, I had an office area in my bedroom. In my first apartment in LA, I used my kitchen.

EveryGirl Extra-Credit Tip: If your bedroom or guest bedroom has to double as an office, then consider buying a Murphy bed—the kind that folds up against the wall when not in use—or a pullout couch.

EveryGirl Extra-Credit Tip: Lack office space? At my last house I converted an outside shed into one. TUFF SHED is a company that will come out and build a shed in less than four hours for two thousand dollars or less. Check rules and regulations in your city or town to see if permits are required.

EveryGirl Office Essentials

Filing System

If you don't have room for a file cabinet, I recommend a plastic file box that you can store in your closet. Your file cabinet is where you'll file all of your bills (carefully labeling folders for gas, electric, credit card, bank, auto, and insurance, as well as one for warranty information on purchased products and corresponding receipts).

I usually extract a previous year's bills and folders from my file cabinet and put them into a box—if you don't have many bills, one of those accordion folders will do. Label the box or folder with the tax year in which those bills were issued and store them. This ensures that I never run out of filing room and that current files are easier to reference. Should you ever be audited or need to refer to an old bill, having storage boxes or folders for each tax year makes referencing a breeze.

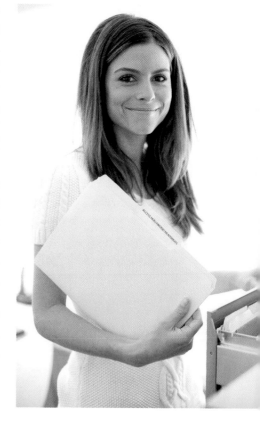

EveryGirl Extra-Credit Tip: To create a makeshift desk, I recommend finding a wooden door (the cheap hollow kind you can get at Home Depot) and resting it on two small file cabinets, or even two sawhorses. If you go with file cabinets, you can secure them to the door with peel-and-stick Velcro. The wooden door provides a large, smooth working space. The desk is easy to break down and transport, too.

Hopefully, your desk will come equipped with a filing cabinet that will have one or two smaller drawers for sticky notes, pens, a stapler, Wite-Out, stamps, paper clips, envelopes, batteries, flash drives, etc. Remember to stock up on extras of these as well. Personally, I look for a file cabinet on wheels, with one large drawer for hanging files and one or two smaller ones for the assorted items mentioned above.

To keep these drawers from becoming junk drawers, I use cheap small plastic bowls and Tupperware storage containers to separate and hold the items.

FILE, DON'T PILE

Apply this simple rule, and paperwork will be so much easier to locate, reference, and access. Items are far better off in hanging file folders than in random piles.

Day Planner

If you can't afford a BlackBerry or other such Personal Digital Assistant (PDA) or are just resistant to technology, then a day planner might be for you. Some people use both a PDA and a day planner. You'll want one that displays an entire week when open. Use it to jot down everything from upcoming appointments, meetings, and events to people's birthdays.

A FEW DAY-PLANNER TIPS

- Your day planner never leaves the house. Ever! I took one to a Laundromat once only to lose it—along with many important dates and information. From that day forward, I have kept it on my desk until the end of the year.
- Keep your planner open so you can see the entire week ahead. When you sit to pay bills or just surf the Net, you'll be reminded of what has to be done that week and be less likely to miss appointments.
- Companies like FranklinCovey make custom planners. You tell them all of the important dates in your life, including birthdays, anniversaries, and even the day you started your job, and then they print the dates in the binder. It's a very cool way to always remember special occasions.
- Check out Google Calendar. It allows you to input important dates in your schedule and to receive e-mails reminding you of them.
- When the year is over, do you throw your day planner out? Absolutely not! You never know when you'll want to refer to a date in the past. Put the old planner in the plastic file box or accordion file folder with the same year's tax receipts.

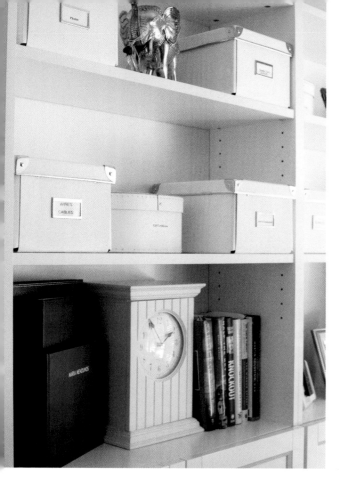

Storage

I have several storage containers in my office closet. I love the color-coordinated ones at IKEA, and Target has great ones, too. I currently have a labeled box for my photos, one for cables (all those annoying cables and chargers that get in the way and that you rarely need), one for receipts, and one for gift certificates. I always used to forget I had them, but now that they have their own area, I don't!

Laptops Are Tops

For your computer needs, invest in a good laptop. The portability allows you to work everywhere—even in front of the TV. They sell minilaptops now with ten-inch screens for under three hundred dollars. They're light and small, making them easy to travel with or tote around the house. If you're a Mac person, the iPad may work for you, too. I love my iPad!

Put old computers that are not fast or lack memory in other areas of your house. I have one in the kitchen, which I use to access recipes.

EveryGirl Extra-Credit Tip: Don't set up voice mail on your phone. So many people have thanked me for this advice. Nowadays we have enough to check with e-mails, texts, BBMs, etc. Voice mail is a thing of the past. I feel free!

EVERYGIRL GOTTA HAVE IT: A DRY-ERASE BOARD

I keep one behind my office door to jot down creative ideas, upcoming tasks, or even quotes I've heard that inspire me. Whenever I'm in the office, the board writings refresh my memory and are thus less likely to be forgotten.

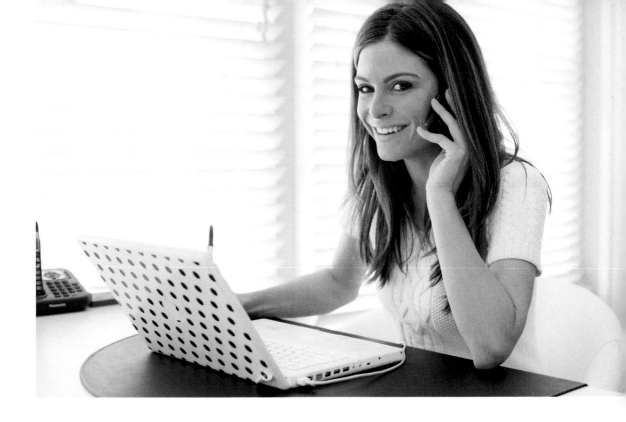

Ask AJ

I am by no means a computer expert. I have all different kinds of computers at home and in my office, from MacBooks to iPads to PC laptops. AJ Jolivette, CTO president, Soho Network Services, Inc. IT You Can Trust, is my computer guru and he has answered some questions on computers for the EveryGirl.

Mac or PC?

Neither system is better or easier than the other. And the common myth that a Mac cannot get a virus is false (viruses just aren't written as much for the Mac, which makes it less susceptible, but you can back up your PC to make it just as virus-proof). Microsoft, Adobe, and other leading companies make their applications for both Macs and PCs. When you take everything into account, your needs will dictate which system is best for you. If you have limited up-front funds, no time to learn how to use a Mac, and financing isn't an option, then a PC is the best choice. If you have a serious "gamer" in the family, then you should absolutely stick with a PC. If you have creative kids with school projects and they want to edit movies, music, and pictures, Mac is the best choice. (Note: If you convert from a PC to a Mac it is VERY important to take a short class at the Apple store or somewhere else on basic use and the differences between a Mac and a PC. Do *not* skip this step; it will save you much time, confusion, and frustration.)

How can I keep my computer free of viruses?

There are a few things you can do to help keep your computer from getting infected:

- Don't click on *anything* that pops up while on the Web, especially if you are a PC user. Remember, Alt+F4 on a Windows computer will close any active window without the need to click anything.
- On a Mac, use "Force Quit." Click on the Apple in the upper left-hand corner; the command to force quit is located there.
- Virus software, of course, is a must. Yes, pay for it, and, yes, keep it up to date, check its alerts, and use it to scan for viruses regularly.
- You also need spyware and malware protection as well.
- Turn off pop-ups and keep them off.
- Don't visit websites to pirate software, get free music, or anything free, on your main computer. If you want to do such things, do it on a spare computer. Those sites are the main culprits for infection and identity theft.
- If you have children or teenagers using the computer, give up on keeping it clean. The best thing to do is let them have a computer to themselves, and keep all financial and other important things off of it, such as family pictures and accounting.
- Keep a restore disc handy. Most computers come with one, or it can be ordered or made with third-party software.

What do I do if I get a virus?

Stop everything. If you are not an expert (or at least advanced), hire an expert. Don't put anything new on your computer, and unplug it from the Internet immediately. It may be necessary to rebuild the computer, so rely on your backups.

How do I back up my data?

RULE 1: If your data does not exist in *three* places, it does not exist.

RULE 2: If you can't restore from a backup, it's not backed up. Test restores on your backups regularly.

Both Windows and Mac come with built-in backup software. Windows backup software is called Backup, Apple's is called Time Machine. You can also purchase third-party applications to back up your data, but remember the number one rule. Your phone is a device, and you should store *nothing* on it solely. *Ever!* All of your contact information, notes, e-mails, and everything else should exist on your computer and be backed up regularly. Your mobile device should *only* be used as a "window" into that data, not a storage place. Just so you know, people *never* listen to this advice until it's too late. Don't be one of those people. However, to back up a BlackBerry device, use the desktop management software that comes with the BlackBerry.

I'm an average gal who wants a good computer. I require basic computer functions like Internet, Word, e-mail, photo storage, etc. What's the best computer buy for my money?

A Netbook. A Netbook is a PC, just smaller, slower, and with limited space, but it will run most applications, comes with a camera, wireless Internet, and is very inexpensive and very portable. Plus, you can video chat and Internet date. The best units are still made by the best companies: Dell, IBM (Lenovo), Toshiba, Sony. Find the one you like, with a nice warranty, and you should be fine. Also, look for these two things: RAM (more than 2 gigabytes), and battery life (more than four hours).

If I want to be able to have an assistant or nanny input info into my calendar via their computer and have it instantly on my BlackBerry, what's the best way to do that?

I would recommend a Microsoft Exchange account to do this. You can order the service on a per-account basis from many different companies. This solution will work cross-platform and is universally accepted for most phones, PCs, Macs, and other mobile devices. Just in case phones break or things change, this solution should always work. However, probably the best cheap way is Google Sync for Mobile. It has shown itself to be a good no-cost solution.

How do I network my computers at home without subscribing to a service?

You can easily get wireless Ethernet adapters and network your home very quickly with a wireless router and very little fuss. Just read the documentation, or hire a one-time installer like Geek Squad. In no time, you'll be sharing printers and Internet. Remember that one infected computer on a network can infect all the rest, so be sure to take virus precautions.

How can I keep my computer clean?

To literally clean the dirt off, use a damp rag and a can of compressed air. Don't use soap and water to clean it.

EveryGirl Extra-Credit Tip: Always try to print in draft mode and on both sides of the paper. This green act will save you paper and ink, time and money.

A Word on Warranties

I buy them on computers and expensive printers, as they're used a lot and are expensive to repair. When I do get warranty cards, I tape them to the back of the products or inside my office closet so they don't get lost and are easily referenced. I also put the code numbers written on the warranty cards on my BlackBerry, along with the appropriate phone number for service if I'm on the road and the product needs service.

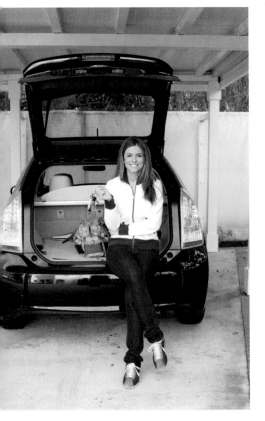

The Car as a Mobile Office

Cruising in my car and listening to music is one of the better ways to clear my head, but I utilize my car as a mobile office, too. I take full advantage of my drive time to make hands-free calls via Bluetooth. I also use my car as a mini closet, desk, and storage area, and as a giant battery, too. With all my jobs—on the red carpet one minute, covering the LA fires the next—I keep extra clothes and makeup in my car to be ready at all times. I keep workout clothes, too, for spontaneous workouts during unexpected openings in my schedule. My friend Harley Pasternak rents out an indoor gym and plays hoops with a bunch of other celebs. When I'm on the west side of town and have an opening, I play.

I also keep a small medical kit—just a good pain reliever for headaches (Excedrin Migraine) and one for other kinds of pain (Motrin), Cold-EEZE zinc lozenges for an oncoming cold or sore throat, and Blistex for chapped lips. Because I have asthma, I store a small portable nebulizer unit—one that attaches to my car's lighter—along with some medication. I've had to use it only once, but when you can't breathe, it's literally a lifesaver. For bad breath, I keep mints and gum.

I also have a phone charging cable and a special AC adapter plug for my lighter (sold at Target) that enables me to plug in my computer to charge or to write when parked. Even though I have a navigator, I have a plastic-coated map of the area, too. It's a great backup if the navigator goes down, and it helps me get a quicker and better physical sense of where I am.

My ashtray is always filled with change. When I get change, whether from a drive-through or from a coffee shop, I put it in the car's ashtray, careful to extract the pennies, which aren't accepted by parking meters. When you get enough forty-dollar parking tickets in Los Angeles, you understand the necessity. I also find a place to keep some petty cash—mostly dollar bills and a few five-dollar bills—to help me out on days my wallet's empty.

EveryGirl Extra-Credit Tip: Please do not text and drive. I've had everyone around me vow not to. I don't want to die texting and I don't want you to, either.

THE EVERYGIRL CAR ESSENTIALS

Have these options and items in your car at all times:

- Navigator
- Bluetooth for phone
- iPod
- AC adapter
- Toiletries kit, including
  - Powder
  - Concealer
  - Blush
  - Eye makeup
  - Lipstick
- Deodorant
- A razor
- Perfume
- Tampons
- TOPSTICK for wardrobe malfunctions
- Flip-flops in case you want a last-minute pedi
- Change of workout clothes
- Almonds

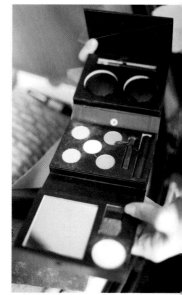

You Are What You Drive

Driving a dirty old clunker filled with trash tells people that your life is a mess and so are you. You need a car that projects a decent image and shows people you're on the path to success. I recommend cars that are green (electric, diesel, hybrid, etc.). Some of the wealthiest people and biggest stars I know drive them. Whether you're eco-friendly or not, you can buy one of those for less and represent yourself well. If you absolutely can't afford a new car, then make sure the one you have has decent paint and remains clean, inside and out.

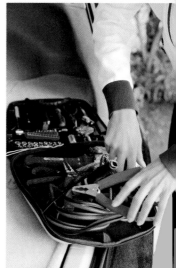

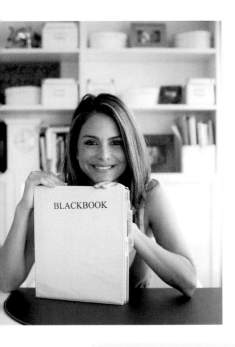

The Black Book

From the time you finish this book to the day you leave this planet, your house must always have a black book. A black book contains all pertinent information in your life. It's an essential reference tool for daily use and for emergencies.

How to Create a Great Black Book

Putting together your black book starts with buying a basic three-ring binder. Then get a variety of inserts, such as plastic sleeves (the kind you can insert 8½" x 11" paper into) and colored separation pages with tabs that can be labeled.

Fill the following pages with the phone numbers and information listed below and also photocopies of bills. My bills do get filed in my office file cabinet. However, I photocopy each one and

WHAT GOES INTO YOUR BLACK BOOK: THE BASICS

You can add categories as you see fit, and more on creating your own black book can be found in the appendix. Just make sure it includes:

- Your emergency contact information, i.e., names and numbers of loved ones and other people to call in case of emergencies.
- Medical information, including all doctors' numbers and addresses, allergies, conditions, prescription information, and parents' and children's medical information.
- Valuable phone numbers, including those for the police, the fire department, lawyers, business managers, dentists, the vet, as well as emergency vet care, the landscaper, the exterminator, the home security company, the plumber, the computer guru, babysitters, dog groomers, the hairdresser, the nail salon, and anyone else who is important to your life.
- Key passwords and pass codes for paying bills or accessing accounts and files.
- Travel information, e.g., car companies, airline information, frequent-flier information, and hotels you like.
- Insurance company information for home, life, and auto.
- Information and numbers for household utilities, i.e., water, electric, cable, etc.
- Social Security and license numbers.
- All birthdays and anniversaries.
- Notes about children, pets, diet, etc. Personalize it as you see fit.

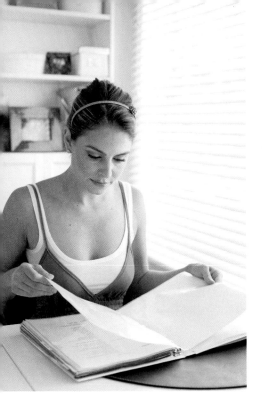

insert it in my black book. On those days when I sit on the phone and dispute some of my bills, add or subtract a service, or the like, I simply open my black book. I then have all the necessary account information I need when asked twenty different times by the twenty different people I get transferred to. Having this information so readily available is also helpful for those times you are sick, injured, or traveling. A friend, assistant, or parent can easily step in and make the calls for you. Your life is so much easier, and the stress just evaporates.

EveryGirl Extra-Credit Tip: Mark down everything you have in your wallet. Write out key information and include photocopies of your driver's license, passport, Social Security card, credit cards, insurance cards . . . everything you would have to worry about if your wallet was stolen. Keep these files in your black book.

Be sure to have a digital version of your black book and e-mail it to yourself so it can remain safely stored in cyberspace. Keep the black book in a private, secure location, too. Check the appendix of this book for more information on creating your black book.

BUSINESS CARDS

You'll also want to pick up another binder and the type of plastic sleeves that hold business cards. I file cards I receive into three categories: friends, industry (those who relate to business), and services (those I hire for auto repair or even hairdressing).

Leave all such books at home. You may think things such as black books, day planners, and business-card holders are antiquated in the age of personal digital assistants, such as BlackBerrys and iPhones. I disagree. The binders are universally user-friendly and won't crash or get easily lost like a PDA will.

PDAs

If you're reading this book, it's most likely because you're someone who wants to do and balance it all. *(Bravo!)* You know how computers have external hard drives to hold extra memory? Well, half of what a PDA can do is be your brain's external hard drive. So many little things—contacts, addresses, passwords, dates, ideas, recipes—can all be easily stored and quickly accessed with one of these cool little devices.

My BlackBerry has much of the same information as a planner. I utilize the calendar on my BlackBerry, inputting meetings, appointments, and important dates and setting the alarm on it to remind me of them and to wake me up in the morning. You can find directions, get information online, and send off quick texts and e-mails, which are faster than a phone call.

They also have GPS capabilities, which not only help direct you to where you're going but can also serve as a means for police or other rescue personnel to find you should you ever have to call 911 in an emergency situation. Being in the news, it's also convenient for me to have a camera on my PDA. Having music on it is great, as it's just one less thing I have to carry.

My BlackBerry is set up so that I, or my assistant, can input things directly into it through a laptop or desktop computer, via programs called Entourage (for Macs) and Microsoft Outlook (for PCs). Any computer technician can set this up for you if it is something you need. For each calendar appointment, my assistant will put who I'm meeting, a quick bio on the person, and anyone else who will be in attendance, the address, and directions. Any and all pertinent information is in there. By inputting the proper information, I'll always get heads-ups for meetings, conference calls, and appointments.

My BlackBerry beeps or vibrates and a message appears on-screen, such as: CONFERENCE CALL WITH JEFF ZUCKER IN 15 MINUTES.

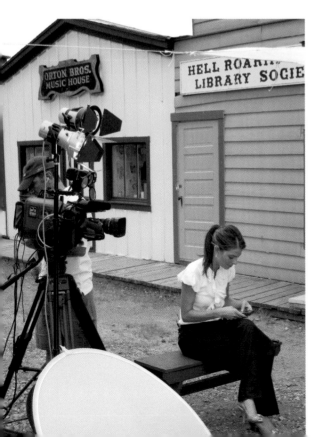

E-mailing my boss while on assignment in Montana, just before my Obama family interview.

Birthdays and anniversaries are also loaded into the calendar, with two-week reminders so I don't forget anyone and have enough lead time to purchase a gift.

In terms of keeping track of my contacts, this is always tricky. I cannot possibly remember everyone I meet, as in my line of work, I meet way too many people. For this reason I input as much information as possible on the contacts—their companies, occupations, trades, or even hobbies. If it's someone who specializes in pit bull dog rescue, I'll input "pit bull rescue" into the line that inquires what company the contact represents. When, say, a year or two later, I bump into someone who wants to adopt a pit bull, I'll simply type in "pit bull," and the name and contact will appear.

GREAT INFO TO STORE IN YOUR PDA

(Be sure to keep a password on your PDA to protect all of this info!)

- Recipes
- Business ideas
- Important pass codes
- Passwords
- Warranty information and codes
- License plate numbers
- Daily to-do lists
- To-do lists for those who work for you, including assistants and nannies
- Crazy ideas you have that could pay off huge in the future!

Under the Tasks application, I type in notes, each with a proper subheading. I have one set of notes in a folder entitled "EGG" for this book. I love the fact that no matter where I am, I can type in any idea that comes to mind. I have editing notes for my movie *Serial Buddies* and story pitches for *Access Hollywood*, *Nightly News*, and *Today*, as well as things I want to ask my doctor next time I see her. My PDA stores passwords, airline phone numbers, mileage accounts, and even recipes. If I go to a friend's house and love a certain dish, I'll type the recipe into my BlackBerry while we joke around.

With the Voice Notes recorder option, I can record something and e-mail it to another person or even send it via Instant Messenger. I also use Voice Notes every time I leave a business meeting, or even my therapist's office, to document what was discussed and what I learned. Again, when you want to do a lot in life, there are things you'll forget, like what you got out of meetings, and it's easier than typing. I suggest it for after doctor visits, too.

With PDAs, you need to do three things: always back up your information and data (I set an alarm on my BlackBerry to remind me), create a pass code to keep your information private, and get the phone-replacement insurance in case you lose it or break it. It's a few extra bucks, but my PDA, and the PDAs of other successful women I know, are literally lifelines. It's organization and information right in the palm of your hand!

EveryGirl Décor

When I started working in Hollywood, I would go to the magnificent homes of the stars and see so little in terms of décor. It was a far cry from what I grew up with—rooms and rooms full of decorations, furniture, rugs, pillows, and draperies. When I did some prodding to find out why the rich and famous had such a bare-bones approach to interior design, the universal answer I got was that many of the homeowners were so overwhelmed with their complex lives, working around the clock and wearing so many hats, that they required their homes to be as simple as possible.

Simplicity in décor leads to peacefulness. I recently visited Kim Kardashian for an *Access Hollywood* interview. It was my first visit to her new home, which was featured on the premiere episode of the fifth season of *Keeping Up with the Kardashians*, and I was blown away. It was so simple, so clean, and so serene. It was the epitome of less is more.

Having fewer decorations means less to buy, which means less debt.

EveryGirl Motto:
In décor, less truly *is* more. Keep clear of trinkets.

I keep the number of display items in my home to a minimum, so the ones I do choose, like this tea set passed down from my mother, stand out.

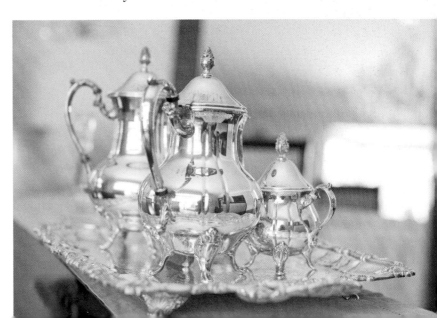

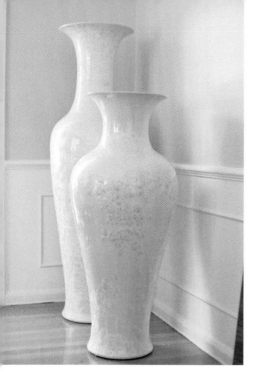

These white vases keep the space simple and clean.

EveryGirl Extra-Credit Tip: Buy a fixer-upper and do it yourself. When the real estate market went down, my houses were still worth what I paid for them because I bought them for less and did the work myself. Have an experienced contractor or friend determine if the house is truly a DIY. You don't want to get in over your head.

There's less to clean, less to get stained or broken, less to replace when styles change, and just less to worry about in general. Trying to look and feel good, to be effective in your career and personal relationships, and to care for your family are a huge order. Going crazy on extensive décor is just another thing to bog you down.

Remember that decorating is an art and a skill that will only improve with practice. I painted my first apartment in the most horrific colors. My dad laughs about how bad he was when he first started working with his hands—he used roofing shingles to panel a wall. Messing up is okay; just stay with it.

Now, let's get into the specifics of how you can buy less but decorate to have an amazing home, starting with finding your home itself!

Get Real About Real Estate

I have a girlfriend who has produced successful films. The problem is that she spent most of her money on high-end shoes, bags, accessories, clothing, and vacations. Today, she rents an apartment and, looking back, wishes she had curbed her spending. If she had, she would own at least one house, if not more. If you haven't already done so, forget the shoes and start saving your money for a down payment on a piece of property. Real estate is the best investment because it's *real*! I don't care if it's a house, town house, condo, or one-room studio—just buy a piece of real estate that you can call your own. It's much better than a closet filled with designer shoes.

My First Piece of Property

When I was first starting out, I had only a three-year deal with *Entertainment Tonight*, so I didn't want to be tied down to a big mortgage. I couldn't get a condo because of my dogs, plus condos don't tend to increase value as much as homes do. I bought a small three-bedroom fixer-upper. It was in a rougher area of LA, but it sat on a flat half acre of land (that's huge in LA), *and* I got it for a low price. With our minds "in possibility," along with many trips to Home Depot and a ton of research, we renovated the property ourselves for little money. The place resembled a mini Beverly Hills estate when we were done, and in fewer than three years the house tripled in value!

EveryGirl Renovations

Doing renovations will make your house newer, cleaner, and more functional, which will make *you* happier, stronger, and better equipped to take on the world. The right renovations will increase the value of your house, too.

Paint

Painting is a relatively easy task and one you must learn. Just applying fresh paint alone when renovating gives any space an instant and cost-effective face-

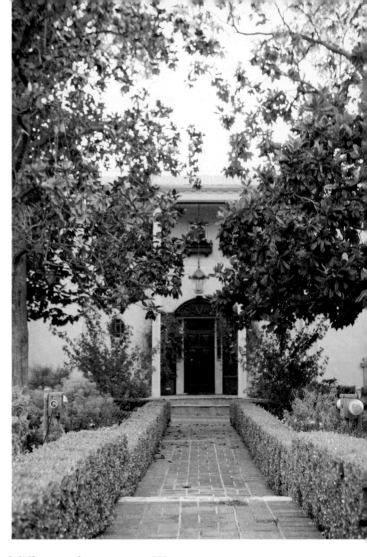

lift. You may want to limit the number of different colors you use. We love simplicity. Also, make sure the color codes of your paint end up in a place that is easy to reference—a basement or garage wall, a PDA, or even your black book—in case you need to mix paint later for touch-ups. And FYI, touch-ups are as easy as taking a paper towel, dipping it into the paint can, and then blotting it on the scratch or nick on the wall.

Have a paint party. My friends Joe Gear and Alyssa Wallerce helped me paint my home in Connecticut.

Latex is a water-based paint that's easy to work with, even if you're not a professional painter. Brushes can be cleaned with hot water and soap. Oil-based paint requires paint thinner and is more

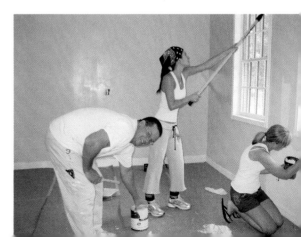

toxic. Oil dries more slowly, too. However, oil does last longer and has a stronger finish that makes scuffs and stains easier to clean. Oil is good for doors, trim, and baseboards, but latex will do the job, too. Semigloss finishes are good for trims, and for kitchen and bathroom walls, as they make wiping and cleaning easier as well.

Renovate Old Furniture

Don't be afraid to paint and alter old furniture and décor. I had a set of natural-wood-stained chaises longues that were not very stylish and rather inexpensive. They had

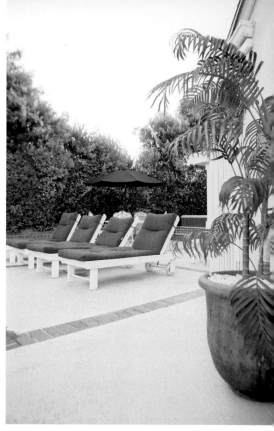

solid-color cushions. Solids, particularly those in basic colors, are always easier to match and have less chance of going out of style. When I moved to my new house, the chaises were out of place, but new ones can cost as much as fifteen hundred dollars!

I researched the furniture you see at high-end hotels. Many of those chaises were white, armless, and sleek. I removed the arms from my chairs by unscrewing a few bolts, lined them all up on top of a tarp, and sprayed them white with an inexpensive power sprayer from Home Depot. It cost about sixty dollars in paint and two hours of work. When I was done, the chairs looked amazing. Welcome to Hotel Maria!

For my kitchen, I was having the hardest time finding a table. I was limited to using something white, due to the other colors in the kitchen. Plus, I had a limited amount of space. In the end, we built and painted a solid white box for less than fifty dollars and then had a glass company cut a big piece of tempered glass with rounded edges to serve as the tabletop. For less than two hundred dollars, I have what I think is the only table that works for my kitchen.

I cannot tell you how many mirrors and frames I've painted or how many pieces of furniture I've broken up to make them work in the places I've lived. You can do the same for your décor. Just have your mind "in possibility" and research online all the many techniques out there for DIY and for designing on a dime. It will save you money, and if you're recycling old furniture, you're doing a little to keep green, too.

Learn from the University of YouTube

By going to YouTube and typing in a home renovation technique or subject that you are interested in doing, e.g., "faux painting techniques," you will get all the information you need. Instructional videos of all kinds will pop up that can teach you not only about décor techniques but also about home renovations of all kinds. I recently needed a sound booth to do voice-overs but knew some cost as much as two thousand dollars. By going to YouTube, I was able to learn how to build one for less than two hundred. If the Internet is foreign to you, then *get to know it!* Ask a friend to teach you about it or go to the local library. There are free computers there to use, and a librarian can show you how.

And Learn from TV, too!

Watch all the DIY shows you can, especially the shows on HGTV. Besides being entertained, there's so much you can learn from them about renovations.

EveryGirl Extra-Credit Tip: Rust-Oleum makes chalkboard paint that enables you to turn a wall into a giant chalkboard. My girlfriend has it in her kids' rooms, but it's terrific for an office, too. Large blackboards or dry-erase boards can cost up to five hundred dollars. The paint will deliver the same effect for twenty.

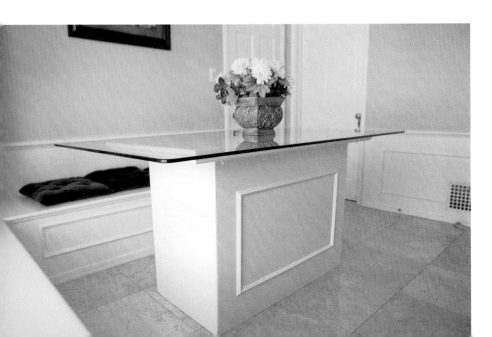

This dining table was made by my dad! The molding makes the table look professional and matches the molding in the house.

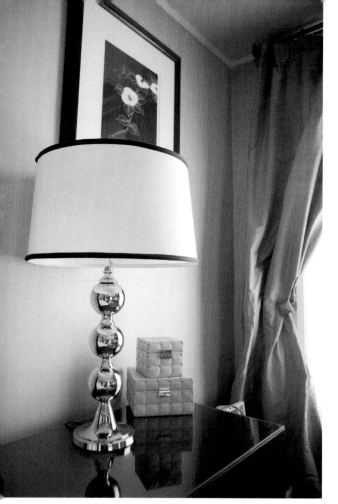

Can you tell that one of these items came from Target? Didn't think so! P.S. It's the lamp!

EveryGirl Extra-Credit Tip: Screwing new sets of knobs and handles to cabinets and other pieces of furniture is a cheap, fast way to revive and renew décor. This technique helped spare me an entire kitchen renovation.

Mix and Match

Another great trick is mixing inexpensive décor with your high-end pieces. I've mixed stuff from Target and yard sales with my nicer furniture and décor. I have a super-wealthy friend who does *exactly* this in her thirty-thousand-square-foot home! I've even picked through a neighbor's trash. They had left out about eight broken screening room chairs. We pulled over with the van, scooped them up, and fixed them. They're in our office edit bay now, and everyone compliments us on them!

Room Renovations

Moving on to more major renovations. Yes, you can do a lot of these yourself or with minimal help. And they will increase the value of your property. There are two important types of renovations that will help make your home worth more.

Most important: The first kind of renovation increases the value of your home. You want to avoid renovations that decrease the value of your home (reducing the number of bedrooms, eliminating the garage, or just decorating in bad taste). Try to keep colors as neutral as possible and limit the use of wallpaper. Future buyers will walk away from a house that needs major repainting or has lots of wallpaper to strip. My parents' house in Connecticut was on the market for so long because it had literally twelve different types of wallpaper.

Renovations should stay in line with the style of the house. For instance, renovations for a colonial home should remain within the colonial flavor. My first house was Mediterranean, so we renovated in that style. Also, it's not good to have one newly renovated room while all other rooms in the house haven't been touched since the Reagan era. Those older rooms will stick out like sore thumbs.

Installing new bathrooms and kitchens will almost always increase your home value, and new windows might not be a bad idea, either. If you have hardwood floors, get them sanded in lieu of getting rugs, which trap dirt and allergens, wear out, and are harder to clean. If you do opt to get your hardwood floors redone, be sure to apply at least five coats of finish for added strength and longevity.

I just heard about the technique of painting hardwood floors on Adam Carolla's podcast (an example of all the free information that is out there). This technique is good for floors that have stains and chips that can't be sanded out. The chips can be patched with wood putty and, after the floor and putty are sanded, you can paint with any color of floor paint you choose. After a coat of primer and two or three coats of your selected color, apply five coats of clear veneer finish. The finish gives the paint permanent protection and the glossy depth that looks amazing.

Second most important: The second type of renovation is the type that makes the home more enjoyable, serene, and fun to live in. Pools, screening rooms, spas, game rooms, outdoor barbeques, gardens, and private areas can save you money, as you'll find yourself, and your family, staying home and enjoying each other's company more.

As I said, my first house sat on a flat half acre, giving us a great palette to work with. We utilized every inch of the property, putting in a spa and constructing a courtyard. It really did feel like a home in Beverly

EveryGirl Extra-Credit Tip: Many of us have parents, friends, or friends' parents who know real estate. Invite them over, show them your list of renovation ideas, and get their opinion.

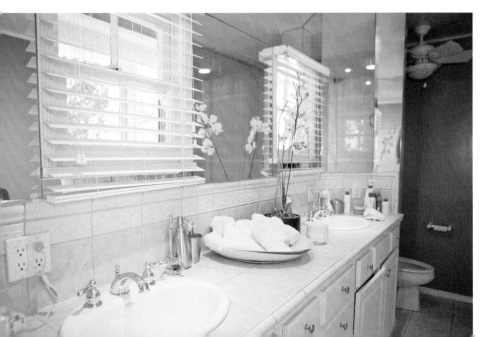

The bathroom is a room to invest in.

Hills. Other show business friends used to ask how we found such a jewel.

We didn't find a jewel; we created one. When you assess renovations, think about how to maximize the space you have. Challenge your brain and pick the brains of people you know who are good at that kind of stuff. You'd be surprised what you can do with an empty corner of the yard, an extra closet, or your basement if your mind is "in possibility."

Meditation gardens, koi ponds, or screening rooms don't have to be out of reach. If you're willing to do the research and the work, none of the above cost as much as you think *at all*! They aren't the amenities for just the rich.

My friend Susan Cabana created a theater for her children. She built a stage in her unfinished basement! The stage is simply a platform built with two-by-fours and plywood and painted black. She painted the walls black, bought red curtains at Target, and put up some clip-on spotlights. Using her old clothes for costumes, Susan's kids and their friends create and act in their own plays after school and on weekends. What an original, creative, and productive use of space that's healthy, constructive fun for the entire family.

Below are listed some of the things that I've done in my house renovations and that you can do, too. Hopefully, you'll come up with new ideas of your own.

In the back of the garage was a small room. We transformed it into a screening room.

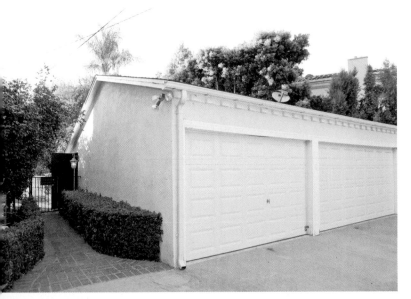

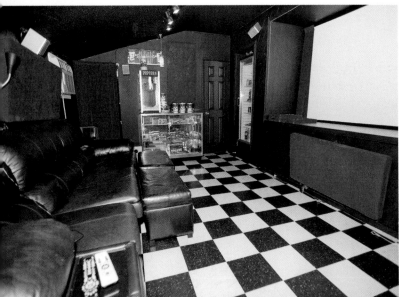

Screening Rooms

Having a great place to watch TV is very important for me. Anyone who says all TV is crap hasn't watched TV lately. Shows like *Mad Men, Breaking Bad*, and *Damages* are some of the best-written and well-acted narratives ever created. I've opted to create a screening room to watch television. For the same price as a large flat-panel TV, you can do the same.

Back in the day, screening rooms meant installing huge projectors and a film vault to hold reels and reels of film. Purists, like director Quentin Tarantino, still use these types of screening rooms, but today, all you really need is a digital projector, a home theater sound system, a DVD player, a white wall, and a space to call a screening room.

Experts will tell you to spend upward of $70,000 on the equipment when all you really need to spend is $625. Projectors can be purchased for under $500. And you can have movie-house-quality 5.1 surround sound, too. (This simply means having five different speakers projecting five different sounds.) For about $125, a home theater sound system, complete with DVD player and the five speakers, will deliver this effect right to your home. It also plays AM/FM, too, for music listening.

You can, and probably will, plug a satellite or cable or both into this receiver for TV viewing. You don't need much space, either. My screening room is literally a rear storage room in my garage. My last screening room was an old shed we converted.

Experts will also advise you to spend $10,000 for a projection screen. Instead, I spent $200 on what they call "screen paint." It has reflective qualities and it's amazing, but I'll let you in on a secret: my parents' screening room in Connecticut is way bigger than mine. Their twelve-by-eighteen-foot screen is merely a wall of white paint, and the image is stunning—zero difference from mine or any other screen. (Mom and Dad's screening room is just a legally converted two-car garage, by the way!)

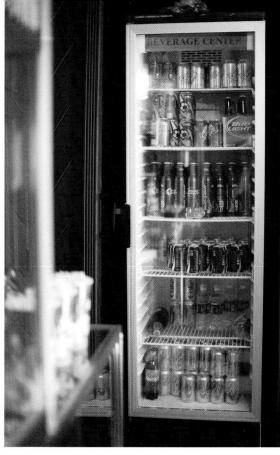

We always keep the fridge in the screening room stocked with drinks to enjoy when watching a film.

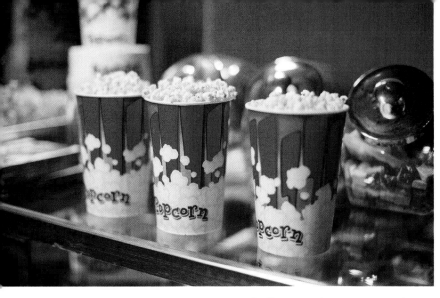

I painted the room black and threw in two pieces from an old sectional couch that my dogs had torn. To accent the room, we made some acoustic sound panels out of foam and red fabric and I picked up a glass candy counter and popcorn machine on Craigslist. The money and effort I put into my screening room has paid off immensely. I use it practically every weekend and it gives me the opportunity to relax after a crazy week.

EXTRAS TO ADD TO YOUR SCREENING ROOM

- An old-fashioned popcorn machine
- A glass candy counter
- Vintage movie posters
- A nacho machine, a sno-cone machine
- A glass refrigerator
- A microwave
- An espresso-and-latte maker

At the end of the day, rather than spend as much, if not more, on a flat-screen TV and a DVD player, I strongly advise you to spend $625 on a projector and a sound system for your very own screening room. Yes, it's still a lot of money, but it's an overall investment in your mental health. High-definition television is just awesome to watch on the big screen. Plus, it's cozy and fun for you, friends, and family, and it's cheaper than going to the movies. The darkness and extra space provided by basements make them excellent locations for screening rooms.

Game Rooms

I don't have children yet, other than my doggies, so what would be a den or family room to someone else has become my game room. Game rooms are great and, like screening rooms, can be pretty simple and cost-effective to create. People in warm climates even have them outdoors!

EveryGirl Extra-Credit Tip: Display old awards you may have received or college or sorority memorabilia in your game room. Don't be shy about framing an old sports jersey of your own!

EveryGirl Extra-Credit Tip: If you live in a warm climate and have a smaller house, consider transforming a carport or overhang into a game area. There are pool tables built for outdoor use.

My game room contains a pool table (it cost me less than $500), a bar (this was already built in, but you can find stand-alone ones for as low as $150), a beer fridge (we Boston girls love our beer), a stand-up arcade machine, a card table (my mom painted an old round table), and sports and movie posters.

My heart belongs to my arcade machine. I've loved Frogger and Ms. Pac-Man ever since my days of cleaning the Channel nightclub back in Boston. I used to play them with quarters I found on the floor. Today, I can play Frogger and Ms. Pac-Man whenever I want, for free! These individual machines cost as much as a thousand dollars each, but I bought a machine that looks just as cool *and* plays not one vintage game but one *thousand* vintage arcade games! I bought mine from a company called Dream Arcades.

Check out sites like eBay and Craigslist for used gaming supplies such as pool tables, arcade games, card tables, dartboards, and other supplies as well. If you have a guy in your life, a game room is something he'll love and a place that he and his guy friends, or you, he, and other couples can have fun in. It's the perfect place to hang up his or your sports memorabilia, too. Don't be afraid to maximize your space and combine your game and screening room, either, as my parents did.

MUST-HAVES FOR YOUR GAME ROOM

- A pool table
- A Ping-Pong table
- A card table
- A dartboard
- A stand-up arcade game
- A PlayStation or Wii
- A couch to collapse on after all that playing
- A minifridge, if you want

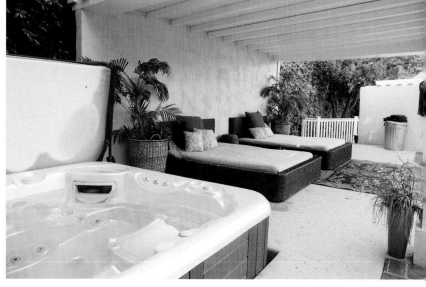

I bought the daybeds at IKEA.

Spas

Experts argue that spas don't increase the value of your house, but I disagree. I feel that luxuries like spas are sometimes that extra nugget that hooks potential buyers. If that's not good enough, then look at it as an investment in your health. Forgo one vacation to have a medicinal tool like a spa that will recharge you daily and fortify you to be happier, healthier, and more effective in your life and career.

Spas are an amazing year-round way to get a good massage and to decompress. I use mine a few nights a week.

Many of the finer houses in LA have built-in spas right next to their pools. The problem is, while elegant, they are made of tile and concrete, with flat concrete seats and jets that shoot water out in a manner not specifically designed to properly massage you. If you buy a stand-alone spa from a company like Hotpoint or Jacuzzi, then you'll get one with seats that are contoured for your body. Moreover, each seat will most likely have a variety of different types of jets. There are jets to concentrate more on the lower back, others more on the upper back, and others for feet.

My feet kill me from standing in heels for fifteen-hour days, and I get pains in my upper back from them, too. We all have different aches and pains, but whirlpool spas help to ease them. I'll get into the benefits of massage later in the book, but you definitely receive similar results in a spa.

You can use it in the morning by setting the jets on full blast. This invigorates you for the rest of the day. Or soak in the spa after a workout or before bed. In my bathroom, I have a heavy terry-cloth robe that I use when I venture outdoors to use my spa. It's southern California, but it does get cold out here, too. Plus having a comfy robe feels good, which only helps me to relax further.

EveryGirl Extra-Credit Tip: When buying a hot tub, bring a bathing suit to the store and try the tubs out. The configurations of the seats and jets are all different and a matter of preference. If you have a partner, bring him along to try the tub out with you, as his opinion will count, too. It makes choosing more fun, as well.

EveryGirl Extra-Credit Tip: Ask the spa pros about specific jets for your unique issues. Mention that you have backaches, or maybe you need stronger jets because you run, ski, etc.

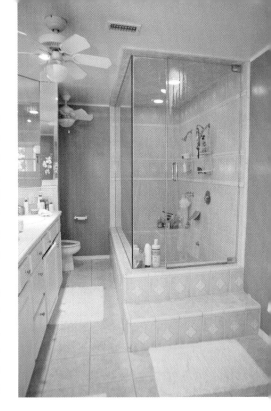

**EveryGirl Extra-
Credit Tip:** You'll need
an electrician to hook up
your spa. This money will
be well spent because you
don't want to make any
mistakes. Depending on
where you live, you may
need to get a permit, too.

**EveryGirl Extra-
Credit Tip:** Hot tubs
can be installed and used
outdoors year-round even
in cold areas. They're also
great in basements and
family rooms. You can get
some tubs for as low as
two thousand dollars.

**EveryGirl Extra-
Credit Tip:** Be careful
with young children
around spas, as they
can easily drown in them.
Keep an eye on pets, too.
My German shepherd
jumped in once!

Spa Alternatives

If it's more convenient, you can have a whirlpool bathtub put in your bathroom in place of your tub. They can cost as little as a thousand dollars. The small drawback is that you'll always have to fill it with hot water and the water will lose temperature in time. Plus, the jets may not hit the body parts you desire.

There are also showerhead jets that shoot water up and down your spine, massaging you in the process. Jacuzzi sells them, with prices starting at a thousand dollars. They claim the jets can be installed without a major remodel.

Steam Showers

My house had one of these when I bought it. I admit I wasn't all that into it at first, but then someone told me it would be a natural way to help my breathing when my allergies flare up. The steam clears my nasal passages and my mind, and the sweat is good for ridding my body of toxins.

The benefits of steam therapy have been known for four thousand years. Some people say that your skin can actually act as another kidney and sweat out as much as 30 percent of your body's toxins. Steaming up will help ease aches and pains by breaking down the lactic acid in your body, and studies show that steaming before bed can treat insomnia. It's also great for skin.

My steam shower is an older unit made of tile and glass, but newer units come in packages that are much cooler. Steam Showers Inc. sells a steam shower for under a thousand dollars that fits into the corner of your bathroom. The showers can also come with body and foot water massagers, fold-down seats, *and* sound systems!

What an investment!

Saunas

Another way to get your sweat on is with a sauna. My old neighbor Margie converted the back of her garage into a sauna. Deciding on whether to install a sauna or a steam shower is just a matter of preference. Do you like dry heat or wet heat? Saunas provide dry heat and can fit into sheds, garages, and even closets.

Just search online for "self-contained saunas," and you'll find many units for under a thousand dollars that will fit into most room corners and require little work in terms of installation.

Chapels

Danielle Weeks, a friend of mine who also stars in *Serial Buddies*, took an empty extra closet and decorated it to be a quiet place where she can pray and meditate. You can do the same. I have another friend who turned a small shed into a chapel. He has an altar and a few pews that he found online, too—just like in a church!

Having chapels on properties was popular on many old Southern estates, and I know a studio president who has one in his backyard. But again, you don't need to be a studio head or have an estate to build your own temple, mosque, or meditation space—you just need to get creative with space and have that mind "in possibility."

Don't worry about the next buyer of the house not wanting a chapel. When all the accoutrements are removed, it's a great office, gym, tool room, or playroom.

EveryGirl Extra-Credit Tip: You can buy portable steam showers for as little as two hundred dollars, and they don't require professional installment. Look online for these if you don't have the money or space for a full-size one.

EveryGirl Extra-Credit Tip: For aromatherapy, you can add essential oils to your steams. You'll find a nice variety at Whole Foods in their cosmetics aisle, in scents including rose and geranium. You can also put these oils on your showerhead to make your bathroom smell delicious.

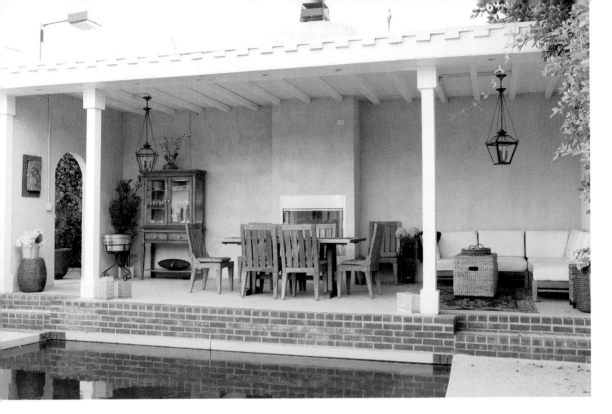

Outdoor Dining Areas

An outdoor dining area works not just for cookouts but also for high-end dining, Sunday brunches, or hanging out with friends. Plus, it provides a nice change of scenery without you ever venturing outside of your front door.

Of course, living in a warmer area enables you to eat outside more. However, you can adjust your outdoor dining area to be used in late spring, summer, and early fall, too. Just like restaurants, you can use propane patio heaters, sold for under two hundred dollars each, for those colder nights.

My outdoor dining space has three walls and a fireplace. I keep dishes and plates out there, along with a dining room table. There's even a plug outlet, high on the wall, for an outdoor TV. There are TVs made to sustain outdoor conditions and project through the glare of sunlight. I know friends who have them, but in all honesty it's just not in the budget right now for me.

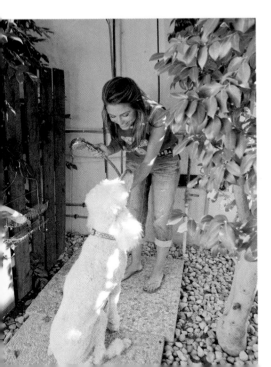

My big babies cost seventy dollars and up to groom. With my outdoor shower, I can bathe them myself!

Outdoor dining areas don't have to be this involved at all. My parents have a simple overhang—four wood posts and a roof. It's probably about two hundred dollars' worth of materials but it is all they need for dining. You can surround this kind of structure with shrubs for shade and privacy (my parents have grapevines) or hang flower boxes around them. Home Depot and Lowe's have great books on how to build these structures, and there are companies that will come out and build them for you for under a thousand dollars.

Vegetable Gardens

All you need is a four-by-eight-foot section of your backyard to have an amazing vegetable garden. You can build a wooden box to raise the garden off the ground, to reduce bending, and also to give the garden a cool look. If you have pets, like I do, you may want to add a white picket fence to surround it, but you can add benches, statues, and fountains, too. The best thing about having a vegetable garden is the healthy benefits. You always have fresh vegetables on hand for cooking and consuming, saving you time and money and ensuring that your produce is chemical-free. Tending to the garden is also a lot of fun. I pick from mine in the morning, making salads to take to work, and at night for dinner. I am eating so much healthier as a result and find myself staying in more to cook.

EveryGirl Extra-Credit Tip: Ceramic fountains are a soothing addition to any backyard. They're simple to set up (in most cases you need only a tiny inexpensive pump), easy to maintain, and not as expensive as you think. The sound is so calming, and it drowns out any noise you don't want your neighbor to hear.

EveryGirl Extra-Credit Tip: Name your garden after loved ones who have passed. A small brass placard can be inscribed with the loved one's name at any trophy store for about ten dollars and attached to a wooden bench, fence, or trellis.

EveryGirl Extra-Credit Tip: Plant fruit trees in your yard. There are different fruit trees for various environments. Having them on your property is a free source of nutrition and decoration. They'll enhance the property value, as well.

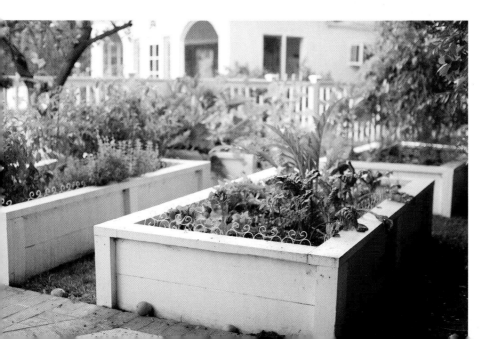

You're the General Contractor

With the boom of stores like Home Depot and Lowe's, doing renovations yourself is much more plausible. These stores not only have all the tools and materials, but on weekends also offer free instructional seminars that teach you everything from painting to laying tile to gardening. Even if you don't end up doing the work, it's great to know how the work is done, making you less apt to be taken advantage of by dishonest contractors.

Internet research will tell you what you should be paying contractors for their hourly rates or what they should charge per square foot, et cetera. Heck, you may even find comments online about the specific contractor you may hire. There are also experts on the Internet who charge as little as fifteen dollars to offer advice in these matters. You just have to use the search engines to find ones that are reputable. I happen to like justanswer.com.

FAVORITE HOME-REMODELING BOOKS

Here are some of my favorite decorating books:
- *Domino: The Book of Decorating*
- *Water Gardens* from *Better Homes and Gardens*
- *Building Screened Rooms* from *Sunset*
- *Outdoor Kitchens* from *Better Homes and Gardens*
- *Home Landscaping: California Region* from Creative Homeowner
- *Use What You Have Decorating*
- *The Find: The Housing Works Book of Decorating with Thrift Shop Treasures, Flea Market Objects, and Vintage Details*

Finding Contractors

The general rule is to get estimates from at least three contractors before hiring one. References from friends and acquaintances are important, too, and whoever is hired should be licensed and insured. Make sure all the work you plan on having done is in a contract. List everything you expect the contractor to take care of—including trash removal, if any.

The price for labor and materials will be in the contract, along with a payment schedule that forces the contractor to be accountable for his work.

A Maria Moment

My old neighbor Margie was, and is, a successful, wise, no-nonsense, hands-on woman. She and her husband, Al, were quietly very successful, yet incredibly modest. She taught me so much about renovations, about being a working woman, and about life.

I'll never forget having her over to show her all of our renovations. When I began telling her about all the other renovations I wanted to do, Marge sat me down for a talk I'll never forget. She told me that I don't need to have everything *right now*. Life is better when you have things to look forward to and dream about—and the bonus is more money is kept in the bank.

Even though I am so blessed to have so much in my life and really don't need anything else, I hold deeply what Margie said. From renovations to jewelry to cars to purchases of all kinds, you don't need to have it all now. Leave stuff in life to look forward to and call them future dreams.

You should also get contractors to sign some form of liability release that releases you from *them* being able to sue *you* should *they*, or their workers, get injured while working on your property.

I usually pay contractors in three to four installments, each installment according to the amount of work that has been done. I've made the mistake of paying contractors for three-quarters of the work when only a quarter was done. I ended up waiting for a long period to get the rest done. By the time they did finish, the work was done to my dissatisfaction (or we would have to finish the project ourselves). Before a contractor receives his last check, thoroughly inspect the work and the property.

EveryGirl Maintains

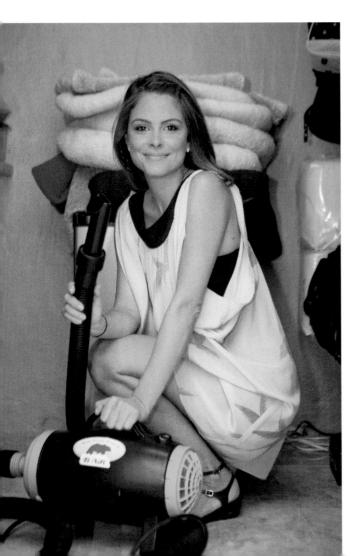

Our early checklist is complete. We have great places to live, work, and plop our pillows at night. Our clothes, cosmetics, and files are where we need them, but unfortunately, the work doesn't end there. We need to maintain this foundation by remaining organized and being clean, too.

The EveryMaid

Let's talk a little about cleanliness. I know I said earlier that clutter was worse than bathroom scum, dust, and mold, and maybe it is, but if so, then filth is a close second. It will surely cause your foundation to erode. My friend Linda Gear once told me what her mother told her: "No matter how poor you are, you can always afford soap and water." By keeping living areas clean, you will feel so much better. You can start by doing one major cleaning of the house.

Cleaning

You can do cleaning weekly and make it fun and productive, too. At my last house, I did my housework on Saturdays, simultaneously doing laundry and paying bills—"stacking" my day. I'll explain more about the effectiveness of stacking days shortly, but let's stick to cleaning for the moment. I would take a bucket with all my necessary cleaning supplies, as well as my dust mop, cleaning rags, and vacuum. Most important, I'd have my iPod going. With these items in tow and with music blaring from my headphones, I would go from room to room, cleaning as fast as I could, setting records for time, dancing, singing, and burning calories like a lunatic in the process.

As a young girl, I would do the same thing when cleaning nightclubs with my parents—except then I got to mop in my Rollerblades. I'll talk more about my days as a janitor later. For now, the point is that cleaning in this manner is a stress-relieving workout that leaves me with such a great sense of satisfaction, too.

As far as products go, I'm using more green, less toxic cleaning supplies these days. But I realize we all live in different worlds and must do what is best and most convenient for each of us. The poisons in some of the store-bought cleaners can be harmful to children and pets. I use vinegar and water to clean all my floors, and I also use Seventh Generation products. There are countless other healthy green products to choose from, too.

I don't do the full cleaning in my house anymore because I truly don't have the time, with work. However, my cleaning person comes only once a week. The lady who owned the house before I did had full-time cleaners seven days a week. The reason my cleaner needs only six hours, as opposed to sixty, to clean the same house is because I "maintenance-clean" and "maintenance-organize" every day.

EveryGirl Extra-Credit Tip: During times that I know I want to deep-condition my hair, I'll take a cleaner and a scrub pad to the tub and shower walls to wipe off soap scum and grime. While food is baking, boiling, or roasting in the kitchen, I'll use the downtime to clean what pots, bowls, and utensils I can. Cleanup after meals becomes much easier then.

Laundering Like a Pro

- Don't throw your clothes on the floor when you undress. Put them back in closets or drawers if they're still clean, or if dirty, toss them in the hamper.
- Positioning your hamper in close proximity to where you undress makes it easy to toss clothes from your body to the hamper.
- Have a bag close to the hamper for clothing that's dry-clean only.
- Buy a mesh lingerie wash bag for dirty hosiery, bras, and underwear. Keep this bag close to the hamper, too. The bag protects your underwear and makes separating and folding time faster and easier. When it's filled, zip it shut and toss the entire bag right in the washer and dryer.
- Keep a bottle of Spray 'n Wash Laundry Stain Remover hidden next to your hamper. For clothes that are stained and soiled, spray the spots and *then* toss them into the hamper. Pretreating means the stains will probably come out. (This is also helpful because you won't miss any stains.)
- Do the wash before the hamper is overflowing. By staying on top of laundry, the task becomes so much less daunting, physically and psychologically.
- Look into laundering services that pick up from your house or work and do the laundry each week for you. There are also laundry services that charge by the pound and allow you to drop off your laundry for them to launder and fold for you. If you find a place like this near work and you drop off and pick up the same day once a week, the cost may be worth it. The time saved may be of incredible value.
- Pick one day a week to always bring clothes to the dry cleaner and one day to pick them up.
- For dry-clean-only clothes, just as with normal clothes, feel free to wear them more than once before cleaning. This will save you time and money. Also be as careful as possible not to wear them where you know they'll get dirty or you'll be sweaty.
- Wash clothes and towels in cold water. I learned this at Earth Day 2010 while working with the "Future Friendly" program, and so far it has worked very well. Doing laundry in cold water preserves your clothing better and saves a fortune on your energy bill. It's great for the environment, too, as it saves up to 80 percent of the energy used in every load.

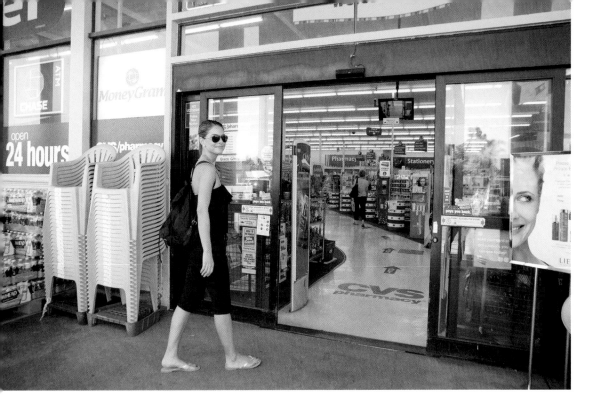

My local CVS is part of a plaza where I complete most of my errands.

Routine

The reason I'm able to work on three very different shows, make movies, manage my household and my appearance, and just plain "do it all" is because I follow a routine. Part of the routine is immediately putting clothes and items back where they belong, but it goes further than that. It also means selecting times and days to do the chores and tasks and then sticking to those times and days while maximizing every possible minute. It's about multitasking and about the process of "stacking and attacking" your day.

Stack and Attack

I developed stack and attack when I was at *Entertainment Tonight*. Designating one day a week (the same day every week) to do all chores and errands, I would make a list of the errands and chores the night before. I would "stack" the order of the tasks on the list in a way that was most convenient to "attack" them and get them done.

My typical day to do it was Saturday. I'd have to do laundry, pay bills, food-shop, go to the dry cleaner, deposit checks in the bank, clean the

EveryGirl Extra-Credit Tip: When parking in large structures, I use my camera phone to take a picture of my parking space and my space number. This way, when I'm done with errands and shopping, I can easily find the space I parked in.

house, watch a DVD for work, and work out. Here's where stacking the day made it all possible. I'd get up early, toss in the laundry, then sit at my desk, open mail, and pay bills. (Today, you can pay bills online, which makes stacking and attacking even easier.)

Next, I'd hit the bank as soon as it opened. Previously, I'd been going to the bank or Target during peak hours of business, standing in line for ages, and struggling to find parking. This resulted in so much lost time and added stress!

Back home I'd finish laundry and clean the house. If I had gone out on Friday night, I'd take a nap, then work out. During my workout, I'd watch my DVD. Last, I'd shower and get ready to go out on Saturday night—feeling strong and fresh from the gym and knowing I was free to have a good time because my week ahead was in order.

SNAKE YOUR WAY THROUGH IT

When you go out to attack your stack of errands, do "the snake." Come up with a weekly defined route that "snakes" to and from your house, with all your errand locations along it.

After the bank I hit the post office, the dry cleaner, and the supermarket—choosing to do business and shop at places close to each other—making everything I need available at either one minimall or one shopping plaza. (Before, I was going to the dry cleaner that was located many miles away from everything else I had to do.) Next to last, I hit the supermarket, due to the fact that food spoils, and then I would gas up my car on the ride home, which is often before noon.

Sundays were for sleeping late and watching football with friends—sprinkling in any chores I may have missed on Saturday. I used Sunday nights to prep for the upcoming week. I laid out my Monday outfit, packed up my computer case and my car, too. I prepared snacks for the upcoming week, such as chopped carrots or boneless, skinless chicken breasts in plastic Ziploc bags. During the week, I'd perform maintenance

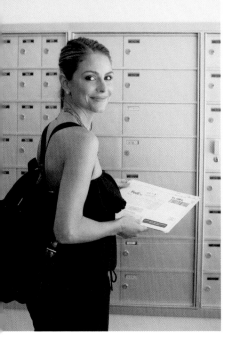

cleaning around the house while cooking or during commercial breaks from favorite TV shows. I'd get workouts in before or after work, too, and also took vitamins every morning after eating breakfast.

There were times I rearranged the order on my list. On those Friday nights that I knew I was going to be out super late, I'd make sure to open mail and pay bills on a weeknight, in front of the TV, leaving only a stack of stamped envelopes to be mailed out on Saturday. I would do the same when I knew I was going away for the weekend. Being more organized, I learned, actually gave me more time to socialize. Until I learned to stack and attack, I had no time for any such pleasures. If I did, it was only because I had swept my chores under the rug. Returning items where they belonged being more organized, having less clutter, and following a weekly routine, I was getting more rest and better nutrition.

At last, my foundation was strong and so was I. I hardly even get sick anymore—knock on wood!

Make a List

When I was first trying to figure out a way to do it all, I sat down and listed *all* of the things I had to do in a typical week—from prescriptions that needed filling down to the face mask that was supposed to be applied once a week. I want you to do the same. If there are things you do monthly, like certain doctors' appointments, then list them, in addition to things you would *like* to be doing in your weeks, e.g., karate class.

Take your time, but be sure to list everything. Keep your list on you at all times

EveryGirl Extra-Credit Tip: I keep inventory lists, too. In areas like medicine cabinets or pantries and even the office, I have a piece of paper in a particular spot with a pen dangling nearby. When, say, the Tylenol runs out, I mark it on the list. Before I go shopping, I grab the sheets so I don't miss anything—saving myself those extra trips to the store. You can find my lists in the appendix.

Ben is a ray of light. When I pick up mail at my PO Box I make friends with the employees who work there. They can really help you out when you're in a jam.

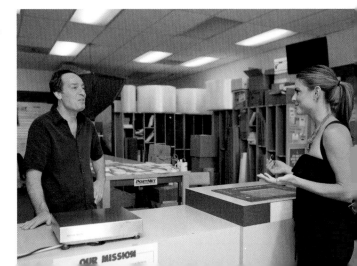

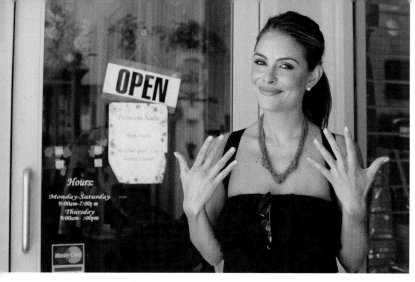

(here's where a PDA comes in handy), then, if you have a free moment, you can refer to it and tick some things off to get ahead.

Create a Schedule

Once you have your list, you can begin scheduling each task and stacking them in a way that's most practical for you. If there's a special face cream that you're directed to apply once a week, do it every Sunday night before you go to bed. If you're taking vitamins (we'll talk about vitamins in more detail in the health section), then take them at a certain time every day, picking the time that's most convenient. I keep my Yummi Bears vitamins by my bathroom sink so I'm reminded to take them every morning when I'm getting ready.

I still try to designate one day a week for bill paying, food shopping, errands, and cleaning. Saturdays are good, but if you have a day off during the week, it's even better for running errands. There are fewer crowds to deal with. If you can't squeeze it all into one day or want your Saturdays to sleep in, then break it up. Do food shopping one specified night of the week, after work, and pay bills or do laundry or both during your weekly viewing of your favorite show.

EveryGirl Extra-Credit Tip: Don't start using a trainer, dry cleaner, or pharmacist located far from your house or your work. If that's not possible, arrange it so they're located in one area. The plaza near my house has a pharmacy, a post office, a pet store, a nail salon, and a dry cleaner! Even better, see if they can deliver to your home or perform the service at your home. In a pinch, I ask my manicurist to come to my house, and it helps save me time.

KISS: Keep It Simple, Sister

By doing errands on only one day and all within one location, we are really just making things as simple as possible. The best way to accomplish a lot *is* to Keep It Simple, Sister.

Stacked, Now Attack!

Creating the routine satisfies only the "stack" portion of stack and attack. The "attack" portion is just as important. I used to dread the minutiae surrounding errands, and that's why I put them off. I just forced myself to be positive about them and to make them fun. Today, I really get energy from accomplishing my tasks, and you will, too.

And Then, Keep Attacking

They say that an idle mind is the devil's playground, and they say it for a reason. Downtime leads to lame time. Lame time leads to boredom, which leads to destructive things. It's during the boring times, when we have nothing better to do, that we gossip, get jealous of others, become depressed, and worse. Keeping busy with constructive things, like your work and your routine, will yield amazing returns. If you keep a daily to-do list on hand, as I do, then making every minute count is a cinch. In addition, whenever you can afford to, accomplish tasks as they come in. When my mother asks me to e-mail her a recipe, it's best just to send the e-mail as soon as she asks for it. To promise to do stuff later and then forget creates stress on all sides. Get it out of the way as it comes in. Never put off things for tomorrow that can be done today.

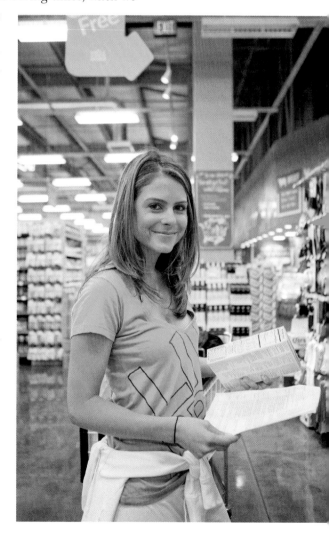

One Day at a Time

As much as you need to have weekly and monthly routines in place and carry a sense of urgency in executing them, take it one day at a time. Simple routines keep stress levels low, but often I'll look at my week ahead and feel overwhelmed and stressed about all the stuff I have to do. I'm learning it's healthiest to stress about only the day you're living—if at all.

Annual Cleanup and Realignment

One of the things I do in maintaining my foundation is my annual re-organizing, purging, and realigning of my life. Some people would call it spring cleaning, but I do this during Christmas week. It's the end of the year, a time when work calms down and most of us get the chance to breathe. I attack every closet and drawer in the house. I go from the kitchen to my office to my bedroom to even my garage, cleaning and reorganizing every storage area there is. In the kitchen, any misplaced utensils are returned to their proper drawers. Tupperware containers are stacked with their proper lids. I attack my bedroom nightstands, my bathroom vanity, and my closets.

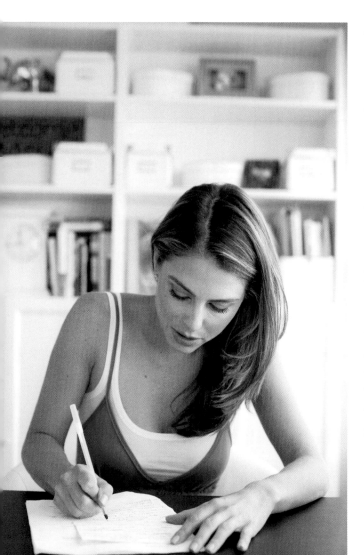

I toss out any old skin- and hair-care products. I shed my closet of any clothes I know I'll never wear. In my office, I go through all my files. Some can be shredded, and others can be boxed with the year's date marked upon it—the technique I mentioned earlier. Junk drawers are realigned—things like elastics, batteries, paper clips, and computer smart drives are all returned to their proper plastic containers. Doing this kind of annual cleaning also reminds me of what I have and where everything is.

If you take the proper steps I outlined to organize your life and you take the proper steps to maintain, then this annual cleanup will be a breeze. I know the last thing you want to do with your days off is more work. I know I dreaded the notion at first, too, but no longer. The annual cleanup during Christmas week helps me to begin the New Year in the best way possible—strong, fresh, and prepared. It will do the same for you.

New Year Plan

The holiday week is also a great time to plan out your upcoming year. I set a day aside, during this week, to create a New Year plan for myself. I write out all of my goals for my career and for my life, as well as events and activities I want to take part in. I do this with someone I can trust for guidance and with whom I can run it all by. Together, we prioritize the order of what's most important to shoot for and what's not worth pursuing at all. It's an official annual company meeting, and I take it very seriously. After all, I'm the CEO of my company, Maria, Inc., right?

But guess where this big company meeting takes place? The mall food court. That's right, one day, every late December, Keven and I meet at the local food court and go over my New Year plan. We sit there for a good many hours, with just paper and pens, jotting down ideas and goals for the upcoming year and how I can go about executing them. The atmosphere and energy is festive and fun—especially when you're not there to stand in lines shopping or making returns. We also have a variety of food to sample, and we do.

Toward the end of the year, compile notes for goals you have or for the things you want to do, and then set an official meeting with friends, family, or mentors whom you trust to run it all by them. If you don't have that person in your life yet, then, girl, have the meeting yourself. You can do it alone. Keep that mind "in possibility." You can always seek out a mentor later.

EveryGirl Extra-Credit Tip: Write down your New Year's resolutions, then seal them in an envelope. You can open them at the beginning of the next year and see how you did. You may be surprised at what you'll see.

A Typical Maria Day (Although No Day Is Typical!)

6:50 A.M.: Wake up with natural sunlight because I go to sleep with the curtains open and often an open window. The night air helps with my asthma, and experts claim a cold room makes for a great sleeping environment. The natural morning light wakes me up gently. I feel refreshed and ready to bounce out of bed.

7 A.M.: I'm out of bed and find my workout clothes right in front of me because I choose them the night before so they're at the ready. No excuses!

7 A.M. to 7:35 A.M.: Work out at my home gym. Maybe I run on the treadmill, do Pilates, or yoga. It depends on my mood. My full workout is written later in the book (see page 176).

7:35 A.M. to 8:15 A.M.: Time for my shower, then I do my own hair and makeup.

8:15 A.M. to 8:30 A.M.: In the kitchen, making breakfast. One of my favorites is half a peanut butter sandwich with jelly and/or banana on sliced twelve-grain bread. Recently, Jillian Michaels turned me on to substituting almond butter for peanut butter, and I love it. Or I love Greek yogurt with honey or a quick egg. I pack a lunch during this time, too, including a turkey wrap with spicy mustard, jalapeños, and a garden salad.

8:45 A.M.: In my car on the way to work, I return phone calls, using hands-free Bluetooth, of course, for safety.

9:20 A.M.: On the *Access Hollywood* set, looking through notes to prep for the upcoming show, arranging interviews, making calls, and having meetings. I also do touch-ups on my hair and makeup.

10:15 A.M.: Get into wardrobe

10:30 A.M.: On the set and taping until 1:30 P.M.

1:30 P.M.: Work meetings; additional shoots; or interviews for *Access Hollywood*, the *Today* show, or *Nightly News*; conference calls, research stories, photo shoots, and movie screenings.

*My days are never the same. I travel about 60 percent of the year, so it's difficult to give a true typical day.

7:30/8 P.M.: Dinner and unwinding a bit while checking the Internet for any breaking showbiz stories. Also playing with my dogs and hanging with Keven.

9:45 P.M.: Watch some reality TV like *Celeb Rehab* or animation like *South Park* as I de-compress and get ready for another jam-packed day.

11 P.M.: Sleep!

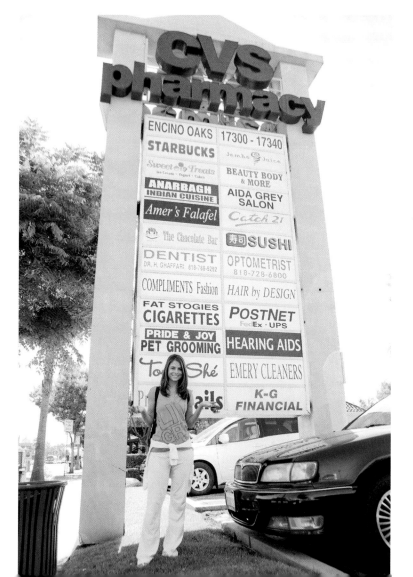

A typical Saturday of stacking and attacking takes place here with a visit to my local minimall. I get my mail from my PO Box, groom my dogs, fill prescriptions and buy any items I need at CVS, pick up or drop off dry cleaning, get a manicure, and eat some yummy Indian food all in one place!

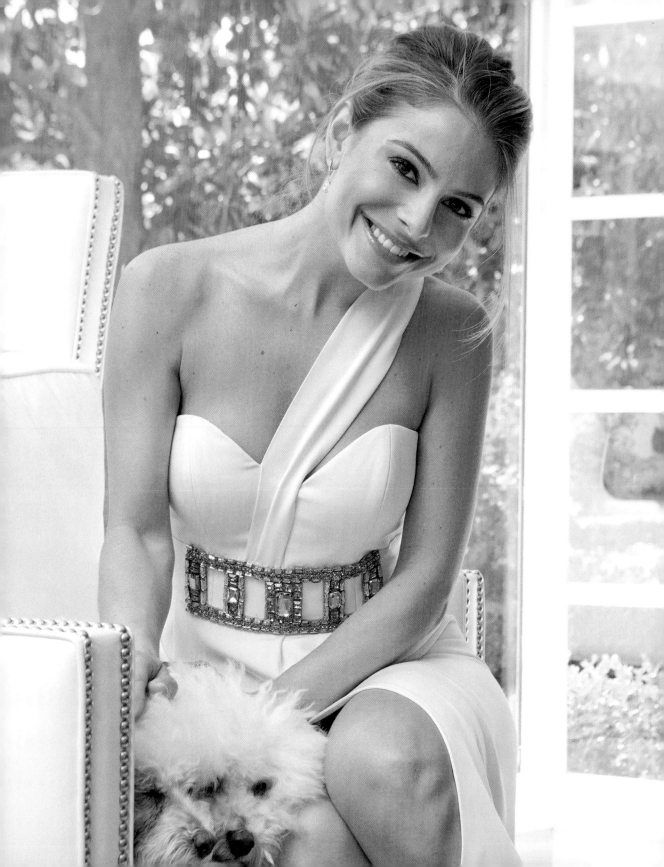

part two

EveryGirl Has Style

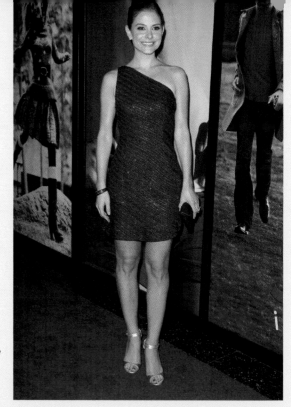

I bought this dress for seventy dollars at a vintage shop.

As I've been saying all along, you're the CEO of your corporation, and every time you're out, you are the number one representative of yourself. Taking healthy steps to look your best will help you immeasurably in life. My working-class father, believe it or not, felt strongly about this, as well, and still insists that I not look sloppy when I leave the house.

In my mind, I am still in many ways the poor girl from Medford, Massachusetts, so I generally remain frugal when it comes to everything, even my beauty supplies. If I have any expensive stuff it's because my various productions pay for them. But there are times that I splurge, too. I use products in all price ranges, and some I even make myself, so you can choose what works best for you and your wallet.

Who better to tell us about beauty than three editors (and my personal friends) of the world's leading publications on beauty and fashion? I asked them which celebrity they found beautiful and why. Their answers inspired me. I'm hoping that, before we get into the subjects of beauty and style, reading their answers will also inspire you.

"I love Beyoncé for her inner strength and outer beauty. Her music, her sweetness, and her athleticism are all things I admire."

—*Lucy Danziger,*
Self *editor in chief and coauthor of* The Nine Rooms of Happiness

"There are so many, but Scarlett Johansson is at the top of my list. She seems so comfortable with herself. Each time we shot her for our cover, she didn't fret about her body or her appearance."

—*Kate White,* Cosmopolitan *editor in chief*

"Meryl Streep is beautiful. Partly because she does not have that 'cookie-cutter' look and also because she seems to glow from within. That kind of intelligence and talent really do make people even more beautiful."

—*Glynis Costin,*
InStyle *magazine West Coast bureau chief*

MARIA'S THREE BEAUTY LESSONS

- No matter how pretty you are, there's always someone prettier, because beauty is in the eye of the beholder. This makes any quest to be the most beautiful girl at the ball a complete waste of time.
- More than anything, someone is beautiful when she has confidence, strength, inner beauty, talent, security, and originality.
- By just smiling and having positive energy, you will become that much more beautiful. Sounds sappy, but really it's true. It works the other way, too. If you always wear a scowl or are a mean-spirited or bitter person, no matter how pretty you are, you will grow ugly.

EveryGirl Skin Care

The healthy meals my parents put on the table when I was younger contributed to a pimple-free complexion back then. But when I went to college, my face started to break out big-time because of all the greasy food I was consuming. It only worsened when I came to Hollywood. The stress, on top of the globs of makeup I had to wear, severely upset my skin. My cystlike pimples were huge. And they hurt, too.

I soon made an appointment with *the* Hollywood skin doc. He gave my face a quick look, told me I needed to buy a batch of *his* skin products (which totaled fifteen hundred dollars!), and then turned me over to his mean assistants, who gave me one of the most careless and painful microdermabrasion treatments ever. I was so desperate to look camera-ready that, even though his products didn't work, I kept going back.

Thousands of dollars later, my former assistant and one of my best friends, Meredith Ahern, swooped in to save the day. Meredith told me about Dermalogica, a company with stores that focus on skin care. Instead of spending thousands, I spent eighty-five dollars, got the best facial, and even left with free samples of products that helped clear up my skin.

Now I have a handle on my skin and know what works and what is just hot air. In this chapter, I'll give you my best skin-care secrets, as well as tips from a few experts.

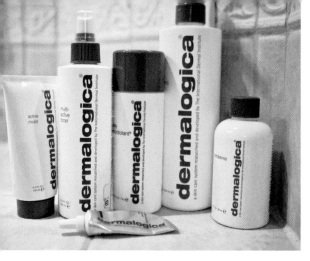

My Skin Rituals

I generally stick to my four-step Dermalogica program below. Now that I'm in my thirties I have added some steps to my evening program. I alternate using different products like serums, collagen-boosting creams, and retinols. One night serum I like is Estée Lauder's Advanced Night Repair. I have also suggested less expensive alternatives to Dermalogica.

Morning and Night

- Cleanser. I cleanse at night with my Dermalogica Special Cleansing Gel. First I use my makeup remover pads (then Neutrogena wipes if I am wearing tons of makeup), then finally, I cleanse with just my hands, no matter how tired I am!.
- Tone. Some toners are meant to remove all remaining traces of oil, makeup, and dirt; others refresh and hydrate the skin while smoothing the surface. I spritz mine on morning and night. My choice: Dermalogica Multi-active Toner or Heritage Rosewater (buy it for a few bucks on Amazon for radiant skin).
- Moisturizer. Without moisture, the skin will not remain smooth and supple. Everyone needs to moisturize. But beware of overmoisturizing, as it can lead to clogged pores and acne. When I'm having a breakout, I use less. I use Dermalogica Active Moist. If you're on a tighter budget, try Colonial Dámes Vitamin E Cream.
- Eye cream. The skin around the eye contains no fatty tissue and is therefore very thin and susceptible to wrinkles. Special eye creams like Dermalogica Multivitamin Power Firm are for-

Makeup-free zone: Working in TV, I have to wear a ton of makeup. My first step to a clear face is removing it completely.

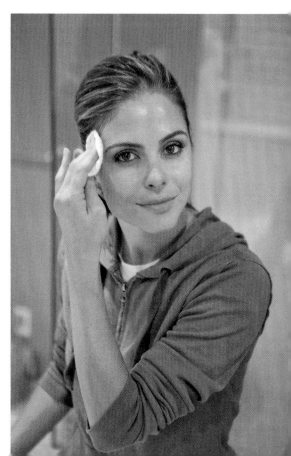

EveryGirl Extra-Credit Tip: Don't use moisturizers with sunscreen at night. The ingredients are not meant to be used 24/7 and can aggravate skin.

mulated to "thicken" this area and reduce the appearance of lines.

- Sunscreen (day only). The number one cause of wrinkles is sun damage, so it's important to use sunscreen from a young age, even in winter and on cloudy days. You can find two-in-one moisturizers that have UV protection for day wear. Or you can rely on the tinted moisturizers that have UV protection I'll mention in the next chapter. Also, I love the sunscreen powder sticks that provide sunscreen in powder form. I keep them in my purse and car for constant reapplication. Many lines carry these powder sunscreens like Colorescience Pro and Peter Thomas Roth.

Every Week

- Mask. I apply a mask once a week. The face masks I like are: Dermalogica Skin Refining Masque, RéVive Masque de Glaise, Elemis Pro-Collagen Quartz Lift Mask, and a homemade tzatziki mask (see pg. 71).

Every Two Weeks

- Exfoliate. Exfoliants work by removing the top layer of dead skin cells that tend to dull your complexion. They also cleanse your pores. My favorites: Ayur-Medic Papaya Enzyme Peel, Ayur-Medic Pumpkin Exfoliant, Dermalogica Skin Prep Scrub, Dermalogica Daily Microfoliant, and fresh lemon.

Every Six to Eight Weeks

- Facial. Whether you get your facial at a place like Dermalogica or have a DIY facial at home, facial time can be your chance to relax and meditate.

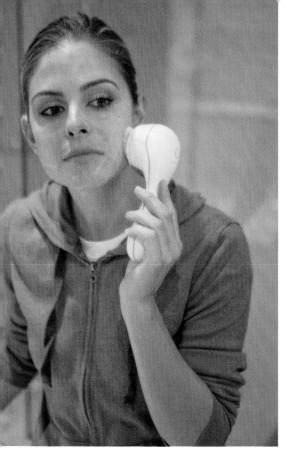
I love my Clarisonic!

It All Starts with a Clean Face

Part of the reason I broke out so badly with acne was that I didn't clean my face effectively. The key is to find a great cleanser that really gets rid of the makeup and grime.

• Makeup-removal wipes, like Neutrogena, help get the day off your face. If you don't want to splurge on wipes that you throw away, buy cheap washcloths and use one per night.

• A Clarisonic Brush takes all the grime off my face and is six times better than regular washing. It's kind of like an electric toothbrush, but for your face. Just charge it up, put a little cleanser on the brush, and then, run it across your face for one minute. You're exfoliating and cleansing at the same time! The machine is sold everywhere from QVC to Amazon, but I found it at Sephora for the cheapest, at $149. It's worth it because you would spend just as much on two spa facials.

EveryGirl Extra-Credit Tip: Always use your face moisturizer on your neck and chest. If you don't want to use your expensive face stuff, get vitamin E cream from your local drug store. It's cheap and effective. You'll thank me later when your neck has been preserved.

"How much is too much product? If you are still rubbing it in after thirty seconds, it's too much!."

—Annet King, director of global education,
The International Dermal Institute and Dermalogica

SKIN CARE FOR ALL AGES

I consulted with one of Hollywood's best skin care experts, Kate Somerville. Here's what she told me about having good skin, no matter what your age.

In your twenties:
- Stay out of the sun. Sun is the number one cause of premature aging. If you are in the sun, wear an SPF of at least 15.
- Establish healthy eating habits. The time is now! A balanced diet will serve your skin well.
- Establish a daily skin-care regimen.
- Please, don't smoke!

In your thirties:
- Begin using vitamin A–based topical products that contain retinoic acid or retinol, which not only stimulates collagen but also turns the cells over to reveal healthy skin.
- Look for products that contain peptides, which add volume and thickness to skin as we age.
- Get facials that incorporate LED lights to firm, tone, and even out the complexion.

In your forties and beyond:
- Incorporate a vitamin C–based product to help brighten pigmentation from the sun.
- Add microcurrent to your facial; it's like a gym for your skin. Those muscles that have headed south are lifted by tiny pulses of electricity.
- This is a great time to supplement with omega-3, which adds moisture to the skin cells during a time when dryness is prevalent.

Maria's DIY Facial

I don't have a lot of time to get facials every six to eight weeks, as suggested. If you do, great, but this is what I do at home in between to maintain.

I reserve my DIY facials for Sunday nights. First I use my Clarisonic Brush for a good two minutes. Then I wash my face with warm water to open my pores, and I dry with a fresh towel.

Next, I exfoliate with either Dermalogica's microfoliant or apricot scrub. I also love the papaya enzyme peel by Ayur-Medic.

After, I open my pores by placing a hot, wet towel on my face. I ster-

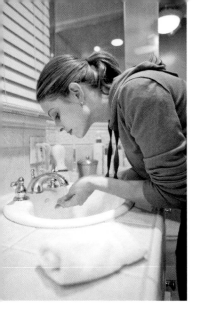

ilize my face with a cotton ball soaked in witch hazel, and then I operate on the blackheads. With my fingers over a clean tissue, I'll squeeze out the blackheads in my T-zone.

I resterilize the area with some more witch hazel and splash my face with cold water to close my pores.

Finally, I apply a mask for ten minutes. Don't neglect your neck and chest. I have recently been paying attention to these areas, and wish I had earlier. I used to think it was a waste to use product there, but it's not. Those areas can never be fixed. Learn from me, and take care of them!

When the ten minutes are up, I remove everything, spray toner on my skin, moisturize my face and eyes, and go to bed!

DIY Facial Recipes

Milk of Magnesia Facial

Ingredients

1 bottle milk of magnesia (unflavored)

Preparation

Apply the milk of magnesia to your face. Wash with a cool washcloth after ten minutes.

My Tzatziki Facial

(or, for the non-Greeks—My Cucumber-and-Yogurt Facial!)

Ingredients

½ cucumber, peeled and sliced

1 tablespoon yogurt

Instructions

Puree the cucumber and yogurt in a blender and apply it evenly to your face. Leave it on for fifteen to twenty minutes. Rinse with cool water and a soft washcloth.

EveryGirl Extra-Credit Tip: Never, ever, ever, ever use a towel more than once on your face. Buy a bunch of cheap washcloths from a discount store like Overstock.com where you can buy a pack of twenty-four for $17.99. One use, and then they hit the hamper. If you let them air-dry to use again, you're growing a science experiment filled with gunky mold spores that you are now smashing into your face. Also, don't towel off your hair first and then wipe your face after a shower. The oil from your hair will go onto your face and create pimples.

EveryGirl Extra-Credit Tip : For a cheap exfoliant, cut a lemon in half and rub it in circular motions all over your skin. The acid helps to exfoliate and brighten your complexion. I walk outside and pick a lemon right from my tree and do this—talk about cheap and convenient!

Dermatologist's note: This can cause irritation and redness on some skin types, so do a patch test before you try it on your face.

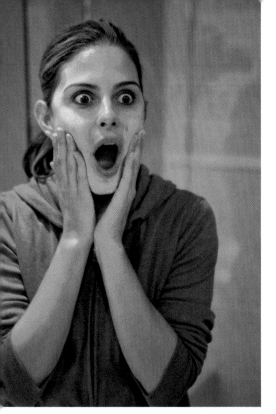

When Pimples Attack

Of course, no matter what you do for prevention, you will sometimes wake up in the morning with a bad surprise. So what to do then? I know people who put toothpaste on pimples to dry them out, which I've tried. It works, I guess, but not as fast as I'd like. If you're looking for a product meant for your skin (and not your teeth!), try Mario Badescu Skin Care Drying Lotion. And if you have serious acne, Proactiv does work. For prescriptions like Doxycycline, which I temporarily used to treat my acne, speak with your dermatologist about all the side effects before finding what is best for you. I also like tea tree oil. Put it directly on a zit and see it disappear.

Nine times out of ten, and I know it's wrong, I pop the pimple with the help of some witch hazel.

Pimple-Popping

First start with clean skin, then sterilize with witch hazel. Be sure to take two tissues and squeeze the zit carefully through them so you don't pass germs onto the rest of your face. Also try not to squeeze hard; the problem when you do is that you open a craterlike area that takes longer to heal. The smaller the hole you burst (whoa, I'm getting gross here!), the better. Then clean with witch hazel again and leave it alone. Another

GETTING RID OF SUN SPOTS

There are two products I swear by:

- DDF Correct and Protect—a moisturizer that helps diminish the appearance of brown spots and contains SPF 15 to help protect from future discoloration.
- DDF Discoloration Reversal—a targeted treatment that helps reduce the appearance of discoloration and age spots.

I've personally seen both work great! If I had to choose one, it would be Correct and Protect.

tip I learned at the dermatologist's office is to wet a little corner of a tissue with witch hazel and affix it to the zit. This helps dry it out. I leave it on at night while I sleep and peel it off the next day.

Skin Care Goes a Lot Deeper Than the Surface

There is so much more to skin care, and to having great glowing skin, than just keeping your face clean, applying products, and popping pimples. You need to make healthy choices in your lifestyle and diet, too.

Avoid

- Processed foods, foods high in chemicals, and carbs, especially sugars
- White flour
- Alcohol
- Too much sodium
- Too much red meat
- Excessive heating or air-conditioning
- Aspartame (a sweetener found in diet soda)
- Smoking
- Recreational drugs

"You can drink and eat your way to good skin care with antioxidant-packed food such as pomegranates, Indian gooseberries, and green tea."

—Dr. Raj Kanodia,
a well-respected international plastic surgeon from Beverly Hills

What to Consume

There are many things we can consume that will help our skin, but just like what to avoid, *it's all about moderation.* Too much of anything can actually be unhealthy. Take it slow. If you're not sure, consult with your physician or a nutritionist.

- Water (Drinking lots of water keeps skin from drying out. It also helps flush out sodium and other toxins. Coconut water is an excellent way to hydrate from the inside out.)

EveryGirl Extra-Credit Tip: If you're breaking out on mostly the phone-talking side of your face, it might be the bacteria that are on your cell phone. Wipe it down with a cotton ball covered in a bit of rubbing alcohol.

- Potassium (found in fish, bananas, poultry, apricots, and avocados)
- Antioxidants (found in blackberries, blueberries, strawberries, pomegranates, and plums)
- Essential fatty acids (found in fish, shellfish, flaxseed [linseed], hemp oil, canola oil, pumpkin seeds, sunflower seeds, leafy vegetables, and walnuts)
- Healthy oils (Oils labeled cold pressed, expeller processed, or extra virgin help keep skin lubricated. You may want to limit yourself to two tablespoons per day, as they can be high in calories.)
- Aloe (found in health-food stores—add your daily dose to water)
- Whole-grains and other foods rich in selenium (found in whole-wheat breads, muffins, and cereals; turkey; tuna; and Brazil nuts)
- Low-fat dairy products
- Green tea (Taken orally or applied to the skin, green tea can reduce the risk of sun damage and help reduce the risk of cancer.)

TAKE YOUR VITAMINS

Vitamins C and E

Vitamins C and E, when combined in a lotion, can help reduce free-radical damage, a harmful by-product of smoke, sunlight, and pollution that causes wrinkles. Colonial Dámes makes a great cream. It's inexpensive and sold in stores like CVS and Rite Aid. Because it's so affordable, I use it on my neck and hands, too. Vitamin E oil is also great for scars.

Citrus fruits and vegetables such as bell peppers, broccoli, cauliflower, and leafy greens are great sources of vitamin C, which helps skin. You can also take vitamin C supplements.

Vegetable oils, nuts, seeds, olives, spinach, and asparagus contain vitamin E, as do supplement pills and oils, which help skin, too. But be careful: large doses of vitamin E can be harmful.

"Every once in a while I spread some pure vitamin E oil on my face. You can buy it by the bottle wherever vitamins are sold. It's sticky, but it gets rid of redness and gives your skin a healthy glow."

—Glynis Costin, InStyle *magazine West Coast bureau chief*

Vitamin A

Fruits and vegetables are loaded with vitamin A, which is necessary for the maintenance and repair of skin tissue.

Topical vitamin A is good at reducing wrinkles and useful in acne control.

Vitamin B Complex

B complex helps maintain healthy skin. A component of B complex is biotin, a nutrient that forms the basis of skin, nail, and hair cells. Biotin is found in many foods, including bananas, eggs, oatmeal, and rice.

B complex topical creams can help give skin a healthy glow and tone, and prevent aging.

Vitamin K

Topical vitamin K creams can reduce circles under the eyes, as well as bruises.

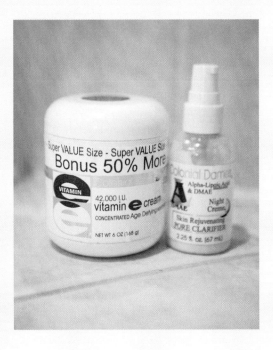

COMBINATION SKIN TIPS
BY EVERYGIRL EXPERT KATE SOMERVILLE

Women tend to have several different skin types on their face. I call them different ecosystems. But women usually use the same products all over the whole face. It's important to treat each area of your face with the products that are correct for that area.

For oily skin

- When you are oily in your T-zone, I recommend getting a facial every six to eight weeks. The pores tend to get impacted with oil, and it's important to clear them out.
- Use witch hazel or a phytic acid–based toner—just in the oily areas—once a day.
- Taking a daily multivitamin that contains the recommended dose of vitamin A is also helpful in controlling excess oil from the inside out.

For dry skin

- Steaming is great for dry skin. If you can buy a steamer or even use a humidifier at night, it will help to add water to the skin cells.
- It's really important to exfoliate. Look for products that contain enzymes, fruit acids, or gentle beads to get rid of the dead skin cells.
- Don't towel off. Put your moisturizer on when you're just out of the shower and your skin is still damp. That will help!
- Taking a fish or flaxseed oil supplement can also help to moisturize the skin from the inside out.

EveryGirl Makeup

Almost all of the celebrities in Hollywood have professional makeup artists who make them up before they appear on camera or even attend events. I was one of these celebs, having been made up, literally, by some of the world's best artists. But hair and makeup took up to two hours of my day. With all the jobs I have, that really inhibited me. So I began doing my own hair and makeup. Today, I can get ready in twenty-five minutes, even less if I have a breaking story. It's just another way I can streamline my life by doing something myself. I do my makeup every day at *Access Hollywood*, and frequently for red carpet events. I'm always proud when I end up in a magazine, knowing I created the look myself! For the cover of this very book, I did my own makeup and styling, too!

The most successful Hollywood makeup artists understand that it's not the amount of product you apply but the manner in which you apply it that truly accentuates and enhances your appearance. Like everything else we've gone over, with makeup, you don't need as much time, money, or product as you may think. It's a craft that you can learn on your own, as I did.

I don't know if any of you caught Jessica Simpson's series *The Price of Beauty* on VH1, but it shed a whole new light on the subject of beauty, at least for me. Like most people, I was conditioned to believe that what is beautiful is what's on

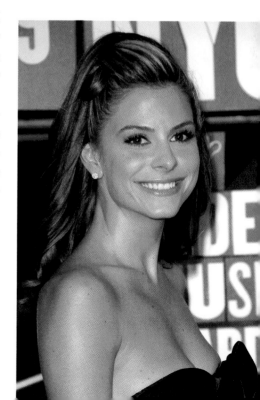

the cover of our country's magazines. Jessica's show clearly illustrated that beauty comes in all shapes and sizes. Different cultures have acutely different perspectives and opinions related to the definition of beauty. Watching the show, I learned there was a place for every look and that beauty truly is in the eye of the beholder. Obsessing to attain the ideal image when there are so many "ideal images" is a waste of time. Be the best that you can be and you will be beautiful.

How I Learned to Apply Makeup

Cindy Crawford was my favorite model and remains one of my style and makeup icons. She's gorgeous, but what impressed me most about her was the fact that her appearance was so natural. I wanted a similar look for myself.

What was particularly astute on my part—if I do say so—was the fact that, in learning the art of makeup, I zeroed in on someone like Cindy, who not only achieved a natural look but also—and perhaps more important—had a skin tone, eye color, eye shape, and hair color similar to my own. I began collecting magazines that featured Cindy, clipping out pictures of her, and hanging them in my mirror.

Every time a new Cindy Crawford cover would come out, I would sit on my floor in front of a mirror and attempt to copy the look on myself using her cover shot as a guide. This is how I learned. It took a lot of trial and error, but I began to get the hang of it. As my confidence grew, I would volunteer to do friends' makeup for school dances and other events. By the time I got to high school, I was a fragrance spritzer at a nearby mall, where I was able to watch the counter girls apply makeup to customers and learn even

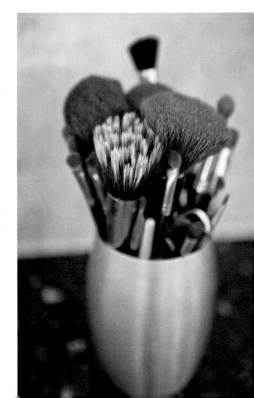

EveryGirl Extra-Credit Tip: Have all your friends pitch in and hire a makeup artist to come over on a Saturday and teach all of you how to apply makeup. For extra, extra credit, hire the artist on a day that you and the girls plan to go out later. The artist can teach you how to apply makeup *and* make you guys up for a night out—all in one session.

EveryGirl Extra-Credit Tip: When getting made up by a pro, whether at home or at a store counter, use a video camera from your phone or a small Flip Video camera to film yourself being made up so you'll remember all the techniques.

more techniques. But I wasn't the only one. Many of the savvier customers would come in and allow themselves to be made up by the counter girls just to learn up-to-date makeup techniques.

Then I Became a Pro!

Anie Spor was the counter manager at the Chanel counter in our local mall. She was a beautiful Frenchwoman who oozed class. She had a sense of style that I had never before seen and was someone whom I knew I could learn from. My cousin Nikki worked for her and we planted the seed with her early on, telling her that I knew how to apply makeup and that, one day, I would love to work for her. Ask and you shall receive. One day the resident makeup artist called in sick, and on a Saturday to boot. I remember pleading with Anie, "I can do this, and you need me." She may not have been sure of my talent, but she most definitely needed me, and so behind the counter I went. I had a blast—making work fun is the only way to work—and by the day's end I had sold a ton of product and Anie was impressed enough to help me land a job at the makeup counter.

EveryGirl Extra-Credit Tip: If there aren't any good makeup artists in your area or they're too pricey, then hit up one of the makeup counters at your local mall. Most of the counter girls know how to apply makeup—many are trained. Bring a picture of a model or actress you want to emulate, and have the counter girl show you which products you need to buy and how to apply them in order to do so. They'll make you up right there. Be sure to have them teach you every application step along the way.

Maria Says

I see many stars who were big in the nineties wearing their makeup today like it's still the nineties! Just like fashion, makeup techniques are ever changing and ever evolving. By flipping through fashion magazines, such as *Vogue, InStyle,* and *Elle,* you can stay on top of what new techniques and styles are out there and have your look evolve with the times. To this very day, I clip photos from magazines to keep up with the trends and to emulate certain looks I admire.

Prepping for and Applying Makeup

Before you put on even an ounce of makeup, be sure to have completed your skin-care ritual, which consists of cleansing, toning, moisturizing, and applying eye cream.

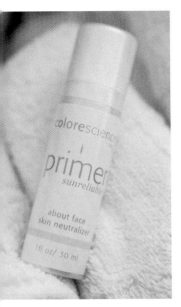

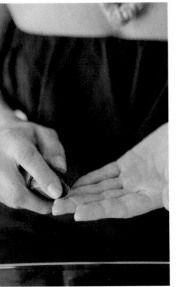

Prefoundation

After washing your face properly, you usually want to apply foundation. But before you do, there's something you'll need to apply first. It's a new step, and I call it "prefoundation"; others call it "primer." Prefoundation is a lovely product that is meant to fill in lines and smooth and prep the skin for perfect foundation application. Smashbox has one called Photo Finish that I like. I also use one from Global Goddess called Upgrade Complexion Face Primer, which actually contains antioxidants and vitamin E, making it good for your skin at the same time. I've used all of them and love them. I also swear by primer from Colorescience Pro, one of my favorites, which I heard about from Cameron Diaz. It's a line tamer and skin brightener. Like the others I mentioned, it makes the skin silky soft.

Interestingly enough, I first tried Colorescience Pro Primer in January and, by April, realized I hadn't had a zit in months. *Odd? No zits? I always get one here or there.* Then I realized that Colorescience Pro is a mineral makeup. The big sell on mineral makeup is that the crushed minerals act as a barrier to prevent the makeup from ever seeping into your pores. The primer was preventing my makeup from going into my pores and clogging them. It not only smooths my skin and preps it for foundation, it also has an SPF of 20 to protect skin from the sun, and it prevents zits! I don't leave home without it.

Foundation

With regard to foundation, you want to pick the one that is the closest and truest match to your skin color. People often make their first mistake here and get foundations that are too pink, too olive, too dark, or too light for their skin tones. We'll use blush and bronzer for coloring, *not* foundation. I have many different favorite foundations. For television appearances, I love Chanel Pro Lumière or Giorgio Armani. They give a nice silky-smooth appearance, but they're pricey. For everyday foundation that's more cost effective, I like: Stila, liquid or

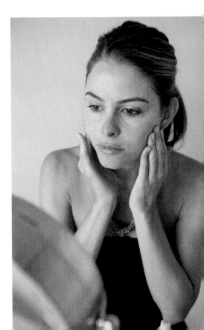

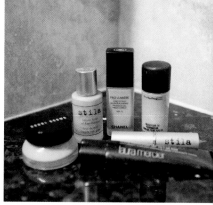

stick (the stick happens to be handy when traveling on planes because it doesn't count toward your liquid allotment!); M·A·C; and for even more budget-conscious ladies, CoverGirl TRUblend foundation. Jake Bailey, who has done lots of my fashion magazine shoots and is the makeup artist to all the biggest stars, like Jessica Alba and Jessica Biel, swears by it. In the end, you really can use just about any foundation. The key is finding the right color and blending properly.

"Splurge on great foundations. Buy different textures and formulations for specific reasons. A tinted moisturizer with an SPF is great for daytime. Use a powder foundation for a quick application and an easy touch-up. A medium- to full-coverage liquid foundation is perfect for a flawless look."

—Bret Boreman, celebrity makeup artist

Tinted Moisturizers

A tinted moisturizer is a combination of a light foundation and a moisturizer. For the ladies with flawless skin or for those who prefer less makeup and a super-natural look, tinted moisturizers are the way to go. Always get one with an SPF to protect your skin. I love Laura Mercier's. It has a nice sheen without looking like an oil slick. I also am obsessed with Bobbi Brown Tinted Moisturizing Balm. It gives you a nice healthy glow without shimmer.

EveryGirl Extra-Credit Tip: My best tip for foundation is to always be sure and apply it to your neck. I often see women with dark made-up faces and lighter necks.

"To give your skin a more natural coverage, try mixing (in your hand) your favorite face cream with your favorite liquid foundation and then apply it to your face and neck."

—Nicole Bryl, makeup artist to the stars, Make-up New York

Application

There are several ways to apply foundation. First and foremost, be sure you are making yourself up in a room with natural light. If you can't

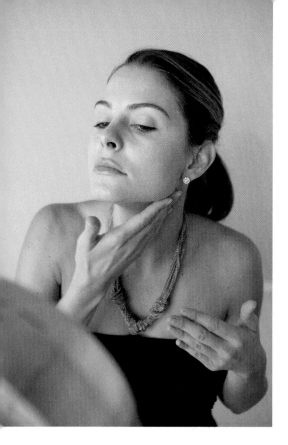

Blending foundation into skin.

use natural light, then use really bright bulbs and take a sizeable mirror outside to double-check all is good! You can use a bronzer brush, a flat brush, sponges, or your fingers to apply foundation. Using a brush applies foundation in a way that gives that dewy look.

My makeup artists Jake and Bret use bronzer brushes to apply foundation. For special events, I'll use that method, too. I squirt foundation onto the back of my hand and dip the brush over it. Then I sweep the foundation over my face, as if I'm brushing it on. Your goal is to make the foundation appear natural-looking, as if a part of your skin. If you do use your hands, then do so *without* pulling on your skin. You want to preserve the delicateness of the skin. Pulling is harsh and leads to wrinkles.

"If you are having problems with blotchy skin, I suggest using a foundation (maybe a little yellow/gold) to neutralize your skin, and stay away from pink or red undertone blushes."

—Mariolga Pantazopoulos,
celebrity makeup artist and hairstylist

ADDING COLOR TO YOUR LEGS . . .

Some people look great pale. I don't feel I'm one of them. So I use Sally Hansen Airbrush Legs. It's sold in places like CVS, and is a great product. It's water-resistant and gives your legs a beautiful glow, or color, depending on which one you buy. I always make sure first to moisturize the body parts I'm about to spray. Then I spray it on and quickly rub in any areas where streaking can occur. It takes moments, and I look golden. I wear it on *Access Hollywood* and red carpets all the time.

Concealers

These are necessary to hide any flaws, such as undereye bags or dark circles. But there are a few tips to applying concealer. Always choose a concealer a half shade lighter than your foundation. Meredith Vieira's makeup artist created a wonderful line of makeup called Eve Pearl. I love her concealer. Another product I love is Colorescience Pro's Corrector Kit. There are a few different colors, in powder form, that treat different problems like redness, as well as blue, brown, and yellow areas on your face. I'll tell you right now, I have not found a concealer I like more for pimples than this. It goes on super soft and stays there. You don't have to work hard at deleting the redness. It's really like magic. There's also a pinkish-red color that removes blue from your skin. On my temples, I have some veins that are really blue. I apply some of this there.

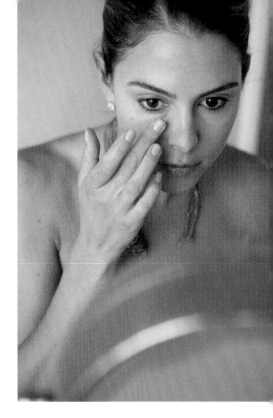

Application

Since a different kind of skin texture exists under your eye, you need to be sure to apply an eye cream before concealer. This will help reduce the appearance of lines and any flaking. The worst thing you can do is apply concealer to dry or flaking skin. It will lie on top of the flaws and instantly age you. *Note:* Eye cream is not necessary if you have already applied a prefoundation, or primer, to your skin. I apply concealer with highlighter mixed into it, using my finger to go just under the lash line and blend it out toward my cheek.

To Hide Dark Undereye Circles

In terms of covering up dark circles, as I said before, the product I'm obsessed with is an undereye concealer from Eve Pearl. Her undereye concealer, in partic-

Colorescience Pro
Corrector Kit

ular, is one I wear every day because it's silky, provides good coverage to hide dark circles, and also highlights under the eye. Most people in my business can't leave home without their YSL Touche Éclat under-eye concealer, which is great, but Eve's concealer gives the same kind of highlight for way less cash.

Dewy Sun-Kissed Look by Jake

We see it in the magazines all the time. Celebs looking dewy, not shiny, as if they just had a refreshing day at the beach. In reality, this look is more because of makeup and lighting than anything else. I asked my makeup artist Jake Bailey how to achieve the dewy glow, and this is what he recommends:

- Use liquid foundation, like Armani, and translucent powder.
- Place a light shimmer (like M·A·C Mineralize Skinfinish) on the apples of the cheeks and top of the cheekbones.
- Use a shimmering eye shadow on the brow bone.

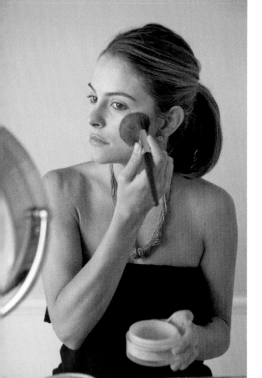

Dust translucent powder over foundation to set it.

Powders

Powder is meant to lock in the foundation and take away shine.

Translucent Powder

One of the best secrets I've learned from working with the pros is using translucent powders. They don't give any color to the skin, which makes for a more natural look. Plus you don't have to go to the trouble of matching your skin color. I wear it on and off camera and currently use Chanel. My makeup artist just happened to order this one for me, but cost-effective ones—from CoverGirl to Revlon—will work, too. I use a powder brush and apply it after my foundation has dried.

Blot Powder

Blot powder is a lot like translucent powder. I have one from M·A·C that I like. Blot powder contains mica and silica to absorb excess oils and reduce shine on the skin's surface.

Sunscreen Powders

There are a slew of face powder sunscreens. I have one by Peter Thomas Roth that I love. It's an instant brush-on mineral powder with SPF 30. It's translucent and beats having to wear smelly sunscreens. It comes in a convenient pop-up tube, and I use it when driving in my convertible to cover my face, neck, chest, hands, and arms. Brush it on all over your skin, and you are ready to go!

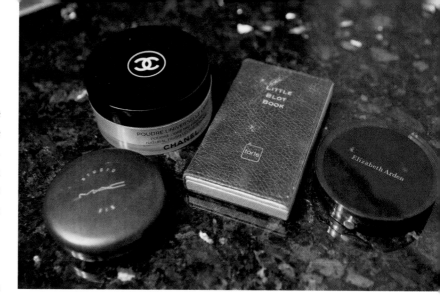

"Faces are like paintings to me; when you look at a painting, your eyes travel through it by following light. In your face, creating these 'light areas' will keep people interested in how beautiful your skin looks, instead of how hard you are trying to cover your dark circles."

—Mariolga Pantazopoulos,
celebrity makeup artist and hairstylist

Bronzers

Bronzer gives the skin a temporary bronzed color resembling a suntan. In my makeup bag, I have two bronzers that I use every day. One is from the Tom Ford Estée Lauder Collection, and it's in Bronzed Amber; the other is from Vincent Longo, in Golden Glow.

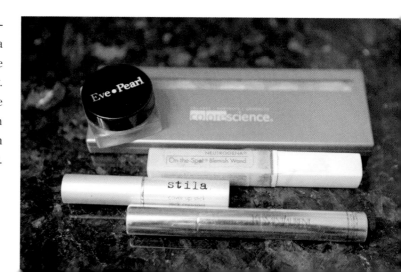

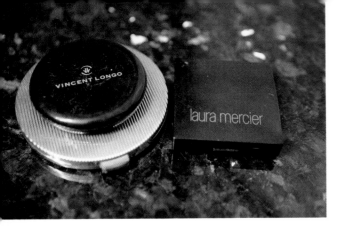

I also love CoverGirl TRUBlend Mineral Bronzer, Natural Bronze 44, which you can find in CVS.

Application

I apply it with a bronzer brush and dust it over my forehead, cheeks, nose, chin, ears (you don't want pale ears and a dark face), and neck. Next, I slowly work the bronzer in, paying extra attention to the cheeks, hairline, and jawline, which is also a good technique to slim your face. Be careful not to get a bronzer that has too much shimmer—that gets to be a bit much. Bret Boreman taught me this technique, as did Nicole Bryl. So don't be scared.

"Avoid applying bronzer in the center of the face, which can make the complexion look muddy."

—Bret Boreman, celebrity makeup artist

Blush

I like to keep a few different colors on hand because blush color has to complement the eye shadows you are working with. So I have peach, pink, burgundy, and so on. In my makeup bag right now is NARS Orgasm, which is a little pink with a little peach; Laura Mercier in Nectar; Chanel's Irréelle Blush; and CoverGirl Cheekers Natural Rose, which looks good on almost everyone!

Application

I always apply my blush to cheekbones, hairline, and jawline. I stroke the hairline and jawline only once and apply just

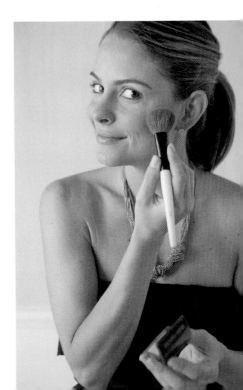

a tad. I also like cream blush, but you have to be careful. You want to make sure to dab it on your skin with a sponge so you don't disturb the other products you've applied (foundations and the like). I've had some makeup artists apply it and make a mess, leaving me with weird lines on my skin. My best tip to avoid this is to spray a sponge with some toner, rose water, or even a little moisturizer and then spread some cream blush onto the sponge and dab it onto your cheeks. Do not wipe or spread, just dab, and you'll love the results!

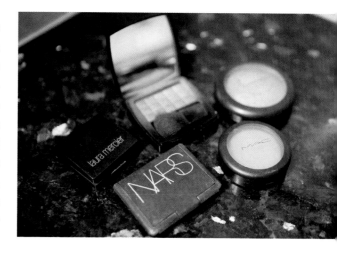

Highlighter

Highlighter is a sheer shimmer that's added over blush to get that J.Lo glow. I love to use M·A·C Mineralize Skinfinish in Shimpagne. It's one of my favorite products because it's a three-in-one: great for eyes, cheeks, and lips.

Application

I apply highlighter to the very top of my cheekbones, just below my eyes, and following the rules for blush, I apply it to the hairline and jawline—just a little though.

A MARIA HIGHLIGHTER MOMENT

While covering the Olympics, I wanted a nude shimmer look for my lips but didn't bring anything with me to Vancouver to achieve that. I experimented and applied the M·A·C Mineralize Skinfinish to my lips with my finger. The results were amazing. It wasn't drying like I expected. It was actually silky on my lips and gave me the perfect color. It also acted like a lip plumper and made my lips look fuller. It's another must-have.

Tanning

I will be honest, I used to hate being pale. I would visit the spray-tanning booth as often as my schedule would allow me. During this past winter, I stopped self-tanning, however. I embraced my whiteness, and it was kind of a breakthrough. But most people love being golden or tan. It always makes everything look slimmer and better. Let me go over your options and how to do each one best.

Lying Out in the Sun

I'm not going to lie; I do lie out by my pool, but since I was in my early twenties, I've used SPF 30 on my entire face and body. My favorite kinds of sunscreen are anything in spray form. Using a spray as opposed to lotions or oils is quicker and neater, and it goes on more evenly. It ensures I won't have weird spots later from lotions not being rubbed in everywhere, too.

EveryGirl Salon Spray-Tanning: Step-by-Step

1. Lotion your hands and feet with barrier cream, then dry off well with a towel—this hydrates them to avoid streaking.
2. Add a considerable amount of barrier cream to the soles of your feet and the palms of your hands.
3. In the tanning booth, rotate your body to coat the inner thighs and the sides of your body.
4. Hold five seconds after the spraying is done.
5. Exit the booth and wipe the barrier cream off your palms and soles of your feet with a fresh towel.
6. Quickly towel dry your face, then your body with another clean towel.
7. Get dressed.
8. Use baby wipes to clean the soles of your feet and your palms only. This will reduce/eliminate orange coloring.
9. Lather your hands and feet completely with lotion, and then wipe them dry up to the ankles and up to the wrists.

Tanning at Home

If you don't have time to visit the spray-tan booth, there are bronzers you can apply at home. Neutrogena makes great ones. Any moisturizer can serve as your barrier cream. Apply it and follow the same steps you would as if visiting a salon. I love Lancome's Flash Bronzer for my face. It smells good and gives a great color.

Self-Tanners

For self-tanners, the kind you apply that gradually give you color, you'll follow many of the same application rules. The best time to apply it is at night. You'll wake up with a nice tan, and won't have that self-tan scent to contend with during the day.

A Maria Moment

Last year, while covering the Academy Awards, I didn't have a makeup artist with me. All that running around meant my face was getting pretty shiny. I didn't have wipes on me, so I used the back of my hand and rolled it over my face. Yes, the skin from the back of my hand blotted up the oil and took off the shine because—guess what? The top of your hand is usually dry, and it's never oily. I pressed my cheeks, forehead, and T-zone and was suddenly picture-perfect. Remember this tip because it will work in a pinch.

Eye Shadow

Eye shadows and eyeliners can be high-end or low-end. High-end products seem to last longer and have stronger pigments. Eye shadows and lipsticks are difficult to resist because new colors are always coming out, and you get so excited you buy them and end up with drawers full of them, like me! When blending these colors, always add layer by layer to control the color.

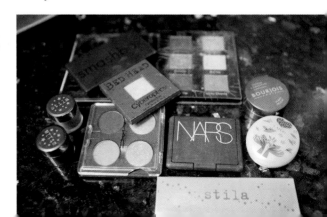

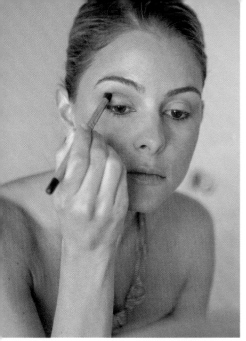

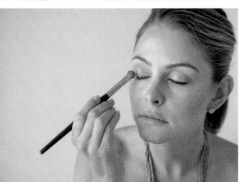

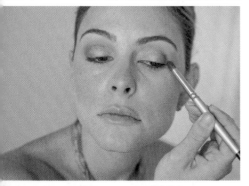

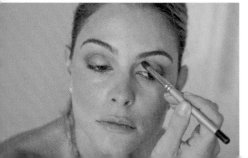

Application

There's really no right or wrong in choosing color. Application is the real key. I've heard experts explain how to do eyes a million times and never really understood them. I am going to attempt to be clearer for you. The difficult thing is that everyone has a different eye shape and different bone structure. Some people have really big eyes; some have small eyes. Some are almond-shaped; some are round. On anything above the eye, like my brow bone, I apply a neutral color or use my blot powder as an eye shadow. You can use either a neutral color, like M·A·C shadow in Shroom, a nice versatile taupe that illuminates the eyes, or L'Oréal Paris HIP Studio Secrets Professional Metallic Shadow Duo in Platinum, which is great for smoky metallic looks on a budget. When I want to apply eye shadow in the crease (the upper crease of my eyelid), I use a brush to apply it in a V shape at the corner crease of my eye.

Applying Cream Eye Shadows

I love cream eye shadows, as well. I use Bobbi Brown Long-Wear Cream Shadow in Beach Honey and Beach Bronze together. I blend the bronze into the crease while leaving the honey on the lid. I use a small, flat concealer brush to apply it and go from the lash line up to the brow bone.

Eyeliner

With eyeliner, I love using kohl pencils, which are mushy and blend well. Stila has a great one in Onyx that I love, too. For a dummy-proof eye, I always go to Stila Smudge Pots. It's my favorite eyeliner because it doesn't move all day. I love it for the inner part of my lower eyelid and even above. I apply it to my inner eyelid rims with a small eyeliner brush and then dust a shadow all over my eyelid.

Aside from Stila Smudge Pots and Stila's regular liners, I also like L'Oréal Paris Infallible Never Fail Eyeliner in black. It's great for a crazy night out because it doesn't fade! Eyeliner

Smoky Eyes 101

My makeup artist Jake Bailey taught me the easiest trick to get the perfect smoky eye. Instead of using a shadow, he recommends lining your eye with a pencil like Smokey Shadow Blasts from CoverGirl or Urban Decay 24-7, and then smudging the pencil with your finger up into the rest of your lid to create a smoky effect.

colors are great, too. I generally use black, brown, or gray. But once in a while, I'll try a bright green, blue, or purple. I also love shimmer liners for fun.

Too Faced has some great kits with colors and a liquid pen applicator. One that I love in particular is called Liquid Eye. It's a shadow collection that, with its trusty liquid-liner applicator, can double as eyeliner. When a product is versatile in this way, it means less money and less product cluttering up the bathroom, too! NARS has great eye shadow combos that I love, as well. Two of my favorites are Cordura and Bellydance. Bellydance pairs a deep, gorgeous green and purple, while Cordura pairs a beige and brown. I use them wet and dry.

Application

I will follow my lash line, as thick or thin as I want, and then use an eye-shadow brush to blend it so the line, yet again, never has to be perfect! That also helps to create a nice smoky look. For extra smoky, do the same on the bottom. To get a sun-kissed daytime look, I start with some blot powder on my eyes, then take my bronzer and dust it over my crease and lid, concentrating more color on the crease. I add M·A·C Mineralize Skinfinish all over the eye, then add a little brown liner to the lash line and blend with some more bronzer, and voilà . . . a nice summer eye. I do this look when I'm on camera, too.

EveryGirl Extra-Credit Tip: When applying eye shadows with a lot of shimmer—and I love my eye shadows with shimmer—take a piece of toilet paper or tissue and fold it under your eye to create a barrier. It will prevent any of the shadow from getting under your eye and creating dark circles you never had!

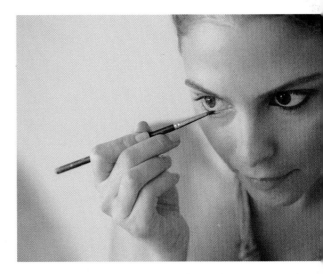

I apply Stila Smudge Pots to my upper and lower inner rims of my eyes.

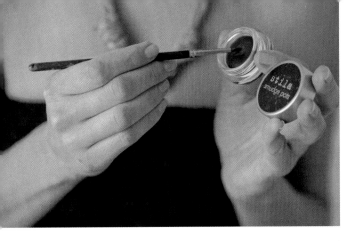

Mascara

If there were only one cosmetic I could wear in life and only one cosmetic I could recommend, mascara would be the one. Great lashes define the most important feature on your face—your eyes. Mascara, when done properly, highlights eyes in a way that inconspicuously lends an overall beauty and distinction to the face. It's a fast, easy, and affordable way to get a great look, and there are so many great cheap mascaras out there. The mascara I've been most obsessed with for years is L'Oréal Paris Vo-luminous. It lengthens and thickens, and it's super affordable. Be sure to replace it every six months.

EveryGirl Extra-Credit Tip: Use a credit card behind lashes when applying mascara to prevent the product from getting on your skin. But be sure and sterilize it first!

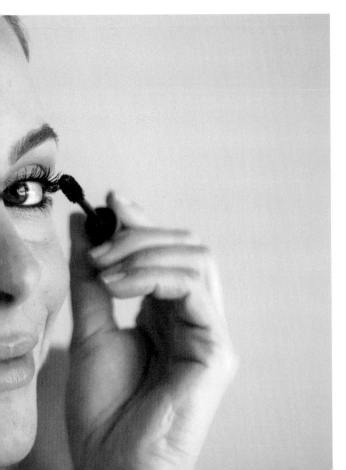

Application

Even when I'm sitting in the makeup chair, mascara is the one thing I always do myself. I feel like only I can get in there deep enough to really lengthen and thicken my lashes. The best way to do it is to bring the brush all the way to the base of your lashes and really work it through. Do it almost as if you are trying to apply mascara to the inner part of your upper eyelid. Sometimes I act as if I'm closing my eye on the brush to really get it in there. When doing my makeup, I spend the most time on my lashes. I really work them and am patient and always apply two coats, one coat ten seconds after the other. Use a good separator if you get clumps.

FAKE LASHES

False lashes are very difficult to apply. Every time I would do my own strips, I would get the "wonky eye" effect—I looked like my eyes were two different shapes. Recently I've learned a few tricks to help. The key seems to be in making sure to wear black eyeliner. This prevents the strip from creating a line that's uneven. Take waterproof eyeliner and line your eye. Don't worry if it's messy because after you apply it, you'll start to blend it upward. This will give you a nice smoky base to apply the lashes to in a fail-proof way. Make sure the band is as close to the lash root as possible. Then, as they are drying, carefully squeeze the false lashes into your lash line. The goal is to try and make sure that the false lashes are one with your lashes.

When it comes to false lashes I usually prefer individuals. I just apply a few with tweezers to the corners of my eye. You can layer a few on there for a more dramatic effect.

EveryGirl Extra-Credit Tip: If you get home and the lashes you bought seem too long for your eyes, don't be afraid to trim them—just be sure and layer one on top of the other so you cut them the same amount.

EveryGirl Extra-Credit Tip: Ladies, if you're not blessed with good lashes, try some of the new lash products that help you get them! Kathie Lee Gifford swears by Rapid Lash. I've seen her lashes and they look like trees—meaning it really works!

"To separate clumpy lashes, use an open safety pin (but do this very carefully in front of a magnifying mirror)."

—Glynis Costin,
InStyle *magazine West Coast bureau chief*

Eyebrows

Years ago I was at a gift suite for the Oscars, and Anastasia Soare, CEO of Anastasia Beverly Hills, looked at me and said, "I've been waiting to get my hands on your eyebrows for years!" I sat in her chair and literally shook as she worked on them. I had *never* let anyone touch my eyebrows. Popi Kyrides, this beautiful woman in my church, pulled me aside when I was in the seventh grade (at the time every girl was waxing her eyebrows super thin, à la Kate Moss) and said, "Don't ever touch your eyebrows." I always listened when I got advice from my elders, and I definitely listened to her.

Anastasia was the first to ever touch them, and to be honest, the entire time I was in her chair I shook, remembering what Popi had told me. I almost cried as she ripped, waxed, and plucked till it seemed there were probably no hairs left and until . . . she whipped my chair around, handed me a mirror, and I saw the results. Her work was nothing short of amazing! It was like everything finally came together. I looked fresh and neat.

Now, with Anastasia's blueprint, I go maybe two to three times a year, doing the in-between maintenance myself. Some women really need to go more frequently, but if you can get away with it like I do, you'll have more time to do the other things in life you need to focus on. Save where you can on time and money.

"Try using a little Anbesol on the intended area before you groom. It will numb the skin and make the whole experience a heck of a lot less painful."

Before I apply my makeup, usually I do maintenance eyebrow plucking and trimming. Then when I'm done with makeup, I fill in with a pencil.

—Nicole Bryl, makeup artist to the stars, Make-up New York

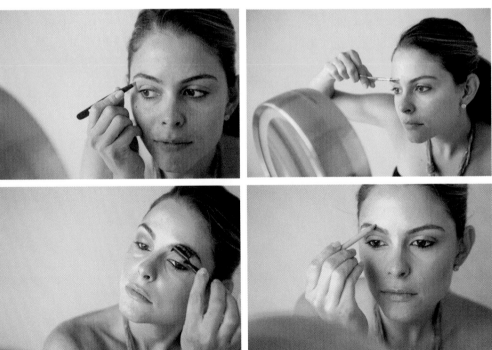

Brow Tips from EveryGirl Expert Anastasia Soare

When it comes to great brows in Hollywood and beyond there is only one name: Anastasia. She not only works on every Hollywood A-lister, but she also has her own DIY brow kit available at Sephora. I asked for her best brow tips.

Q: What are your top three or four steps when it comes to achieving perfect brows?
A: Step 1—Have a great brow kit with stencils to work with. This will eliminate the stress of choosing the right shape and drawing it freehand, as well as balancing that shape on both the right and left brows.

Step 2—Arch your brows in natural light to prevent removing too many hairs. Do this outside or by a window during the day.

Step 3—Less is more. Start with a more natural shape, and give it one day before you decide to remove more hairs.

Step 4—Always pencil or powder your ideal shape on top of your brows and use that as a guideline of where to tweeze if you don't have stencils.

Q: What defines great brows?
A: Great brows should follow your natural brow bone, meaning that a brow arch a half inch higher than your brow bone can be considered way too much.

Q: What can you do with brows that are too light or too dark?
A: Light or very dark brows can easily be fixed with Anastasia Tinted Brow Gel. It's a great cosmetic way to achieve that perfect shade and is easily removed with makeup remover. Tinting can be scary, as brow hairs have been known to turn orange or really dark.

Q: How can women do a quick brow fix?
A: In a pinch, use a pencil and some clear brow gel to achieve a perfect look in less than a minute.

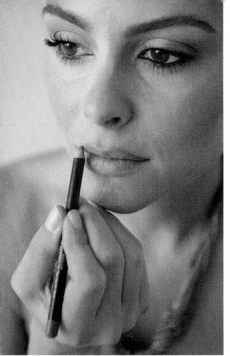

Lips

Nude Pencil

To line or not to line: that is the question. I do both. Sometimes I line my lips for an event or party, but for everyday I don't. I like to use a nude pencil on the lips to avoid showing that I even lined them. We all usually overdraw even a little, unless you are blessed with plump lips, so a nude pencil helps to add without advertising it. Begin by tracing the natural lip line, blending the corners and softening the edges with a lip brush to diminish any hard lines. Add a lip balm or clear gloss.

Lip Glosses

I then usually stick with glosses, as I love them. Stila just came out with a new line of glosses that are kind of matte and don't move. I also love the cheaper brands at CVS. Let's face it: you will always need to reapply, so it makes sense to go with the cheaper brands if you don't have money. The only difference I've noticed is mostly in just the color options and textures.

Lip Balms

Sometimes when my lips are dry, I use a stained lip balm like Hollywood Lips. Bret created the line, and I love it! I also use Smith's Rosebud Salve, too. For stronger healing purposes, I love Blistex and have it by my bedside and in my car.

EveryGirl Extra-Credit Tip: Buy the lip liner you love and use Smith's Rosebud Salve over it as a gloss. But remember to put gloss only in the center bottom and top of your lips.

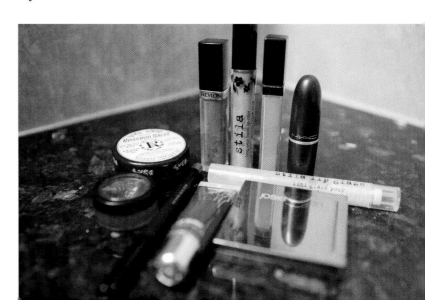

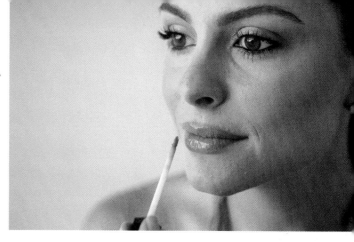

"I suggest exfoliating your lips every day by taking a lip balm in a pot and mixing it with some sugar. Use your index finger to apply the mixture and massage all over the lip area. Remove excess with a tissue. The sugar will gently remove dry skin, and the lip balm will add needed moisture."

—Bret Boreman, celebrity makeup artist

FIVE STEPS TO SEXY LIPS, BY MAKEUP ARTIST TO THE STARS NICOLE BRYL, MAKE-UP NEW YORK

1. Use a good old-fashioned hot wet washcloth to exfoliate your lips if they are dry. The rubbing motion will also help to plump up your lips and make them fuller.
2. With a powder puff, prime the upper and lower lips and outer edges of lips with a dual-finish powder foundation. This ensures a clean slate for the lipstick or gloss or both to adhere to and help the chosen color stand out. (This also helps to prime the mouth so the lipstick, liner, and gloss stay on longer.)
3. Add your lipstick color of choice to the center of your lips only. Liner comes next.
4. For an ultrasexy look, you will want to line your lips *after* your lipstick has been applied. Liner helps to define the lips, makes them appear fuller, and also stops lipstick from bleeding. Applying it after lipstick makes it easier to blend onto your mouth so the actual line doesn't overpower the lipstick. Blot the mouth ever so slightly and *never smudge the lips together after the lipstick is applied!* This only creates unwanted lines on your lips and smears the lipstick over the edges of the mouth.
5. Finally, add a very high-gloss lip gloss.
   Note: You don't need to use dark colors to create this ultrasexy look!

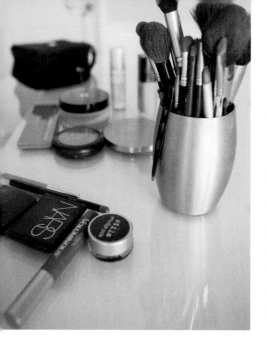

EveryGirl Tools of the Trade

The right tools are essential for any job. Makeup is no different. Can I do my entire face without anything but my fingers? Yes, and in jams I have. But it's not ideal. For the proper tools, you can go as cheap or expensive as you like. I have everything from CVS- to Chanel-brand brushes. I have to say, I didn't buy the most expensive ones. My shows have bought them for me. Cheaper brushes don't feel as nice, and the bristles easily fall out, but they will achieve the same look. If you want to splurge and spend, it should be on the powder and bronzer brushes, in my opinion. Below is a list of my must-haves.

Must-Have Brushes for Your Kit

- Powder brush
- Blush brush
- Bronzer brush
- Three eye shadow brushes
  - Big bristle brush for blending
  - Small pointed brush for crease work
  - Regular brush for applying eye shadow to the lid
- Eyeliner brush
- M·A·C 130 Short Duo Fibre Brush

MARIA'S FIVE-MINUTE MAKEUP ROUTINE

There are days when I have no time to tend to my face. Here's my five-minute routine: Apply tinted moisturizer to the face and neck; add cream blush, which I apply with a sponge, blotting so I don't move the tinted moisturizer; apply some quick powder, and then put on two coats of mascara. Pet the dogs, and I'm out the door. By the way, if I had only one minute, I'd do just the mascara because mascara is everything. I never leave home without it.

Makeup for Darker Skin

I asked expert makeup artist to the stars (including Oprah!) Valerie Hunt for some tips for women of color. Here's what she had to say.

- Avoid using taupe or muted browns because they don't add any flavor to enrich dark skin.
- Lighter-skinned African-Americans (e.g., Beyoncé or Halle Berry) look best in soft peach blushes or eye shadows. Mocha beauties like Oprah Winfrey look best in warm orange and rust blushes.
- Use lip colors that can be rich in either oranges, pinks, or reds, or soft golds, bronzes, and peaches.
- The key to having a polished look is to always wear a warm blush, at least two shadows in gold on the brow line and eyelids, and a rich crease color in burgundy, deep espresso brown, or dark green.
- For more information, check out Val's blogs: valsbeauty.blogspot.com and valsbeautyblog.wordpress.com

Hot-Date Makeup

Most girls never believe this, but guys don't like a girl who is overly made up. I recommend an understated look that's still sexy and gorgeous. My favorite date-night look is a little silvery gray shadow from Stila dusted on my lids; and on the crease, as well as on your eyes' inner rims, the black Smudge Pots; plus, two coats of mascara and some powder blush over the foundation. I'll use a great tinted balm or nude lip color with that look. I hate the idea of reapplying lipstick on a date, so the tinted balm is great because if you reapply it, it's quick, doesn't require a mirror, and balm is for chapped lips, so you don't look vain. You never want to be the girl at the table reapplying makeup.

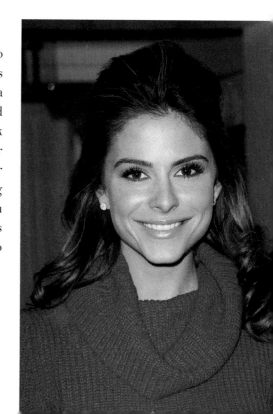

Gym Makeup

Even though you're there to sweat and get in shape, I'm sensitive to the fact that a gym is a place to meet people and that you still want to look your best. Here's a nice compromise: all you need to do is apply some tinted moisturizer to your face, maybe some concealer to any pimples, and waterproof mascara to your eyes.

WHAT'S IN MARIA'S PURSE? SHE PACKS AND TELLS.

This is what I keep in my purse at all times:

- Stila foundation stick
- L'Oréal Paris Voluminous mascara
- One to two lip glosses that I rotate in and out
- Moisturizing lip balm with color
- Blotting sheets
- CARGO face powder
- A small powder brush
- Bobby pins
- Minibottle of hair spray
- Blush
- SPF 30 brush

MARIA'S FIVE FAVORITE PRODUCTS

- L'Oréal Paris Voluminous mascara
- Chanel Pro Lumière foundation
- Bobbi Brown Tinted Moisturizing Balm
- Eve Pearl concealer
- Stila Smudge Pots in black

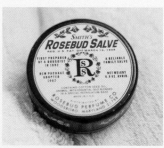

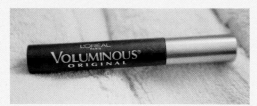

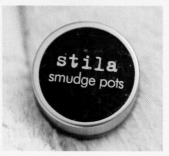

Maria's Red Carpet Looks

This is a fun evening look. Nicole Bryl did this look for me.

I created this simple yet still red carpet glam look.

Use yoru M·A·C Mineralize Shimmer along with your bronzer for this glowy look. Don't forget your Stila gray shadow and Smudge Pots, and L'Oréal Paris Voluminous Mascara.

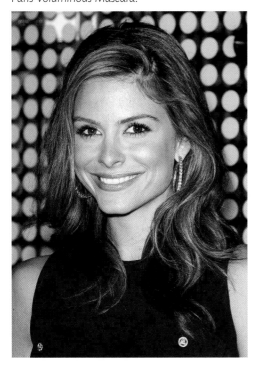

This is a great smoky look Bret Boreman created for the Benjamin Button premiere. We added a lash strip for drama.

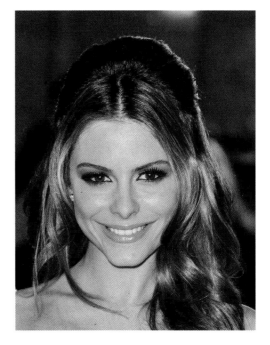

CHAPTER SEVEN

EveryGirl Fashion

The Basics

When it comes to fashion, I try to keep my wardrobe simple. It's hard because being on TV means I need more options. When I wear something and am photographed, the outfit kind of needs to be retired. But most of my stuff is solids, which means I can change the look and make it fresh with different accessories. I have the basics, including black T-shirts, white T-shirts, a leather jacket, camisoles, tanks, cardigans, a good jean jacket, a few great blazers, and some amazing thin little Club Monaco sweaters that are pretty and do all sorts of double duty over both shirts and dresses. (I buy them in lots of different colors.) I have several styles of jeans and a few little black dresses (LBDs). My wardrobe also includes flats, heel, and boots with different heel heights for different occasions.

My best fashion advice is to buy what fits your body and what makes you feel your best. You need the basics, like jeans, an LBD, great plain tees, and a blazer, and then you can change everything else around them. You also need a great trench coat and a basic black peacoat or winter coat. A beautiful coat

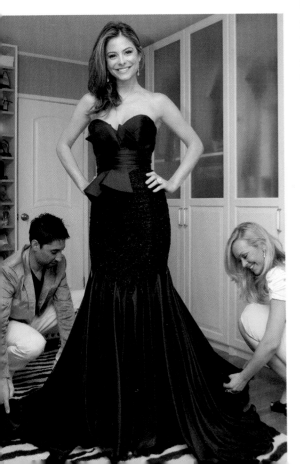

Michael and Tamara of Ralph & Russo adjusting a potential Emmy gown.

will last you forever. When you find that perfect something, buy it in multiples, either in different colors or in the same. Ask the saleswoman if she'll give you a discount because you are buying in bulk.

For basics, my friend and fashion expert Rachel Zalis recommends Theory, J. Crew, Banana Republic, Bloomingdale's own line, and New York & Company. She also hits up H&M as an affordable alternative.

A MARIA MOMENT: THE FASHION EDITION

In May 2000, Channel One News, the place Anderson Cooper started, called me in for an interview. It was the job opportunity of a lifetime, and I had to compete against hundreds of other girls. I knew I had to look my very best, make the right statement, and I had to stand out. But even though I think I have good taste in clothes now, back then I was clueless in terms of styling.

I drove to the Burlington Mall and popped into a Forever 21, where I saw two well-dressed salesgirls. Whether they knew it or not, these two were my very first stylists! I told them I was really in a bind and needed help—that I was up for a TV-hosting job and needed an outfit that said "MTV meets *Dateline*."

Ask and you shall receive.

The two salesgirls jumped into action. Together we came up with the perfect outfit and accessories—colorful and hip yet tasteful. It wasn't a ton of money but much more than I was used to spending. However, this was such a huge opportunity for me that I freely ran the credit card (more on investing in yourself and career later in the book). I flew to NYC, had a great interview, and got the job. And guess what? One of the things that impressed them most was the way I dressed and the fact that I could bring them a style they seemed to lack.

That job launched my career, and the experience proved the impact fashion can have and how easily even someone with lesser means can be fashionable. Now let's get you up to speed with the help of some of my expert friends.

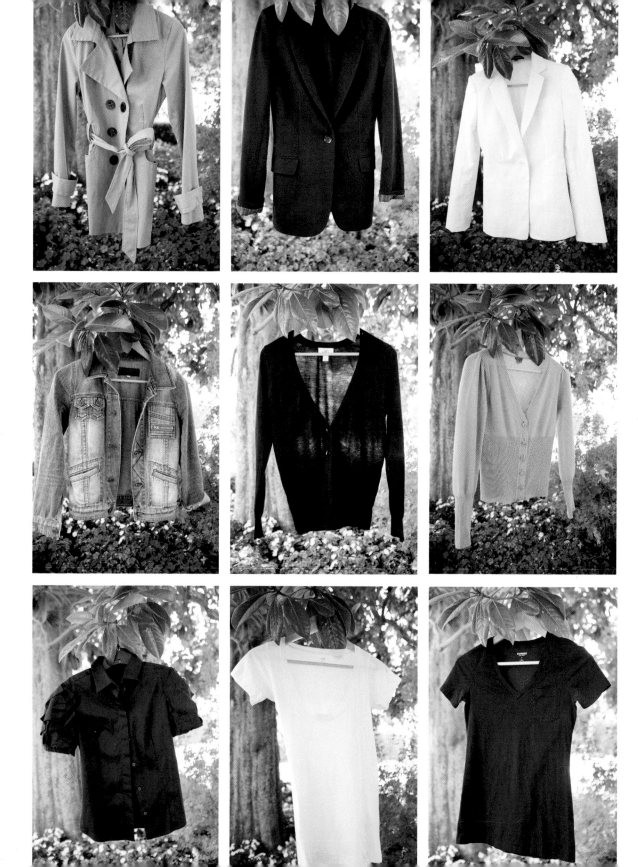

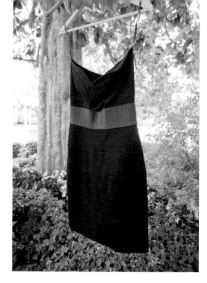
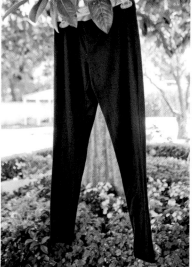
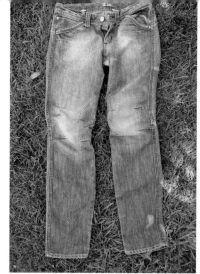

Build your wardrobe around basic pieces like these. They're classic so they will always be in style: a trench coat, a black blazer and a white blazer, jean jacket, black and camel cardigans, black or white button-down, basic black and white T-shirts, a LBD, black pants, and of course, jeans. These jeans are from H&M. They're cheap and I live in them.

My Favorite LBD

I have a great LBD from Caché that I bought back in my days of doing beauty pageants. Yes, I still have it! It's the perfect generic strapless little black dress that's fitted at the knee. I wear it by itself or with a little sweater or a cropped leather jacket. The same black dress, with the right accessories—like a belt, scarf, or necklaces—can be worn in so many different ways.

Color

If you've always been a bit afraid of color and wear only black, take baby steps into the world of color by wearing a colored T-shirt under your black blazer. It's just a tiny color commitment! I know there are many ladies out there who believe that black's the most slimming color, which means their entire wardrobe is this one color. This can get boring, and black is actually aging when you wear it next to your face. Personally, I like to wear colors. In fact, my best friend, Alyssa, laughs and says, "Whenever you come home and I pick you up at Logan Airport, I can spot you a mile away." What can I say? I love to wear yellow, red, and even pink.

EveryGirl Extra-Credit Tip: Revolveclothing.com and shopbop.com are two websites that tell you exactly what trends are in for each season. They show pictures that help you easily identify which trend is right for you and how to wear it.

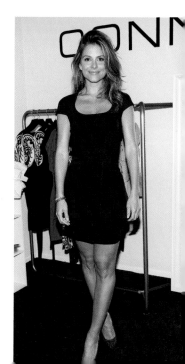

I recently bought this French Connection LBD. It resembles the fit and feel of a Herve Leger and I love it!

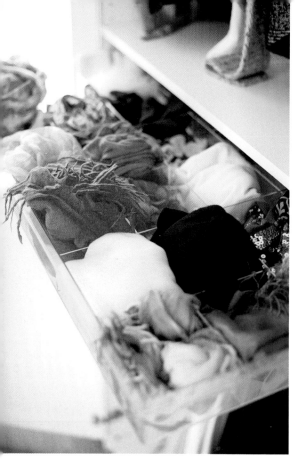

I use bright accessories, like these scarves, to add color to my look.

"Always add a layer or a completer piece. I like to think it's always the third piece that adds flavor to an outfit. A jacket over a blouse and pants, a cami under a sweater, a big colorful scarf over a T-shirt and jeans. It's the cherry on top of the sundae, the piece that pulls an ordinary look into something more styled and deliberate!"

—Stacy London, cohost of TLC's What Not to Wear *and cofounder of Style for Hire*

Size Is Just a Number

Sizes on clothing are all over the place these days. A 31 at H&M can be a 28 at Express. Just buy what fits your body well. Don't get bogged down in numbers. It's better to go a size bigger than have a muffintop hanging over your jeans.

Few of us, if any, have the bodies and skin tone to look amazing in everything we put on. Being fashionable isn't about just being up on the trends. A major component is about dressing to your body type. Is there a part of your body that you don't like (say, your arms)? Don't get stressed about it. (Just don't go sleeveless!) I will never wear a Kate Moss outfit or anything in satin, because they show my every imperfection.

Many times stylists have brought me the most gorgeous dresses (on the hanger) to wear on the red carpet. But if they don't play to my strengths, I won't wear them.

"Don't try to compete with women who are younger and thinner by wearing clothes that don't suit you. Great style is based on where you are in your life at the moment."

—Stacy London, cohost of TLC's What Not to Wear *and cofounder of Style for Hire*

"Bring a camera with you when you're shopping, and have the saleslady take a picture of you . . . from behind!"

—*Rachel Zalis, fashion expert*

Hemlines

I'm not going to get into inches here, but the point is that too short . . . is too short. If you're constantly adjusting and feeling like you're flashing people, then it's just too short. Maybe you have the body to rock that look, but even if you do, don't rock it too hard. It's not about age and body type but the appropriateness of your look. Be proud of your body but not obvious.

Look at stars you admire of different ages. Helen Mirren wears plunging necklines to awards shows, but she covers her legs and arms. She's sexy without going overboard. Jennifer Aniston plays up her assets in a classy way. And to me, that's the sexiest look of all.

Buying High and Low

There are times to spend and times to save. You know me; I will find ways to save as much as possible. But I do realize that it is good to invest in some of the staple pieces I discussed earlier. You want those basics to last forever, to be well tailored, and to outlast the changing trends. Sometimes this means saving up and spending more to get that perfect piece. However, there are always alternatives; nowadays stores like Target, H&M, Urban Outfitters, and Forever 21 are selling lower-cost versions of designer clothing. I have some gorgeous jewelry pieces from Vera Wang's Simply Vera collection from Kohl's. I bought the cutest ankle boots from Target.

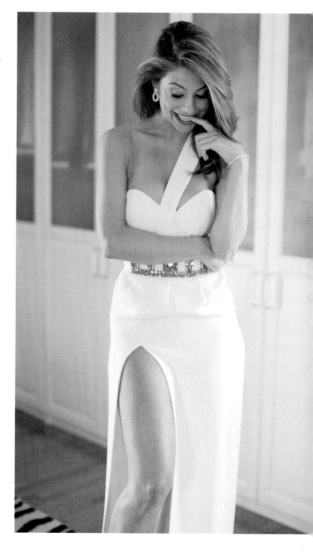

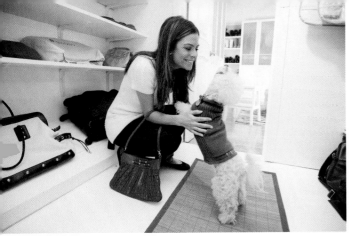

This Treesje bag is definitely a classic style you can use forever. My pup loves it, too!

Where to Spend

If you're going to splurge in fashion, try to stick to the classics that won't go out of style, so you can enjoy them through the years. The classic Chanel handbag, cashmere cardigans, the LBD, pearls, diamond stud earrings, a great trench coat, and a good wool coat.

If you have a ton of money, go for it. Just remember: I'd rather you own a house than a closet full of Gucci bags, and I certainly don't care if a "star" is wearing it, because that doesn't influence me, either. By the way, most people don't realize that stars have been mostly loaned those high-end designer items, including shoes, bags, and jewelry. It works out great for these companies because suddenly Jennifer Aniston is wearing it, and then Jennifer Smith from Ohio buys it instead of paying her rent. Be careful! I have so many friends who don't have a penny in the bank but a closet that looks like they have their own NBC series.

Go Cheap on These Things

Hanky Panky makes my favorite undies for eighteen dollars. However, for the budget-conscious gal Victoria's Secret makes the same kind, three for thirty dollars! H&M has their version for $2.99 a piece. Examine the fabric to see if it seems well made; you can buy that ninety-eight-dollar black Ella Moss T-shirt or one that's a little less soft at the Gap for nineteen dollars—twelve dollars on sale. Splendid makes great tees, but Express makes super-soft knockoffs. It's about what you can afford. There's something comparable for every budget.

Give Secondhand Stores a Second Look

New York and LA have some great stores, like decadestwo in West Hollywood, where stars resell their wardrobe collections, making them available to the public for up to 80 percent of the original cost. I got an amazing Prada shirt for a hundred bucks. I recently discovered a great store in Chicago called Sofia Vintage. They sell old and new stuff, but I was blown away by the quality selection. They go to great lengths to weed out junk and carry only cool stuff. Wherever you live, there are always little gem antique and vintage stores that you can hit up to put a great outfit together. My assistant, Cate, always puts together the greatest outfits, and they almost always come from vintage stores. Her whole outfit usually is less than forty dollars! But be careful not to get carried away and buy stuff that you won't ever wear.

Customize Your Clothes

Sometimes you'll see a great dress but hate the belt because it looks cheap. I see it all the time. I recently swapped out the belt that came with the dress for a gorgeous vintage belt I bought for twenty bucks to attend a big meeting. The women I met with flipped out, and it got the conversation started off on the right foot!

Sometimes we look at an old coat and think, *Ugh, I've had enough of that coat! I need a new one.* If you read the advice of everyone in this section, you'll see the word "staples" come up often. Staples are the things you must always have in your closet that mix and match with everything.

A black peacoat is a great staple, for example. Let's say you've had it forever and you're tired of it. You don't have to throw it out. All you really need to do is spruce it up by changing out the buttons. Get some fabulous gold nautical buttons or shiny silver ones. If you can't sew, your local tailor can, and for little money. This instantly gives the coat a face lift. I know you've probably heard this before, but if you actually do it, you'll do it on all your old clothes. Don't be afraid to tweak outfits and clothes and put your own signature on them. It's also very green of you. I've had the same tan trench coat from Express for years. I too got tired and am in search of the right buttons as we speak!

Accessories

I love accessories because they not only dress up an outfit but they're an easy way to make five outfits out of just a few pieces of clothing. I love shopping for accessories at Forever 21. Always on trend, they have great jewelry, hats, and headbands! Never throw out your old ones, because they will come back when you least expect it. Here's a list of some of my go-to accessories:

- Hats. I love cool hats of all types.
- Long and short necklaces. Even if long or short isn't in, you can still wear one or the other, and you can always layer them. Sometimes I tape necklaces in the back to make them short.
- Belts in all shapes and materials—thin, thick, metal, and leather. Never toss them, because they will come back. It's just a matter of time.
- Good diamond stud earrings. It doesn't matter if they're real or fake. Just be careful with the real ones because you don't want to lose them.
- Layered rings. I love the stackable kind.
- Bracelets of all kinds, including silver, gold, inscribed leather ones, and bangles.

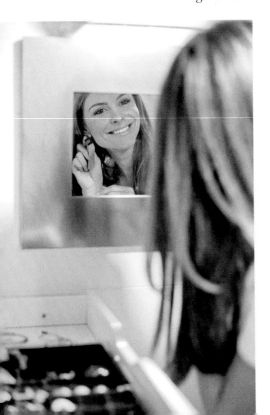

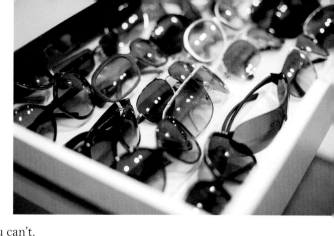

- Good black sunglasses. You can't go wrong with Ray-Ban Aviators. Invest in them, and use them forever. It doesn't hurt to splurge on a great pair of Chanel sunglasses if you can afford them. They will always look cool and help bring luxury to an inexpensive outfit. You can get similar frames for way cheaper if you can't.
- Great boots. I have a pair of Coach ones that really stand up—season after season

THE BACKPACK

You may not think it's as cool as a Louis Vuitton bag at first, but believe me: once you go backpack, you'll never go back! I was in New York performing in the Broadway play *Chicago*, of all occasions. As usual, it was a "stacked" day. I had to rehearse for the play, host segments for *Access Hollywood* and *Today*, get interviewed by other TV shows around town, and attend a few business meetings, too. Normally I carry my purse and a separate bag for my laptop, and I struggle, awkwardly, to get from location to location, and my shoulder and neck end up killing me. Because I was so slammed, Keven got me to condense everything I had into his backpack. *Hallelujah!* The clouds parted. Rainbows formed. I was able to carry all my stuff and move swiftly and comfortably through New York in a way I never had—and without bodily pains and strains. Backpacks don't put the same strain on your body. On the contrary, they keep your back straight and improve your posture. Today, I use a backpack whenever I have too much to carry, and it has helped me so much.

When all I have to carry is my wallet, keys, and lipstick, that's when I enjoy my handbags. My favorite lines are Coach, Treesje, and Linea Pelle. I have a Prada backpack that I bought for about two hundred dollars. There's a company called HandbagCrew.com that sells a variety of them.

I was so inspired that as soon as I came home from New York, with a sense of urgency and with my mind "in possibility," I began meeting with bag manufacturers to create a backpack of my own. If you're worried that backpacks don't seem fashionable, then remember, the same thing was said about flat shoes and look at how popular they are now. I happen to think the right backpack *is* very cute and highly fashionable.

Shoes

Yes, I'm a shoe gal! The twist is I don't wear a lot of heels. I have no threshold for pain anymore, which is why I'm always in flats. Wedge

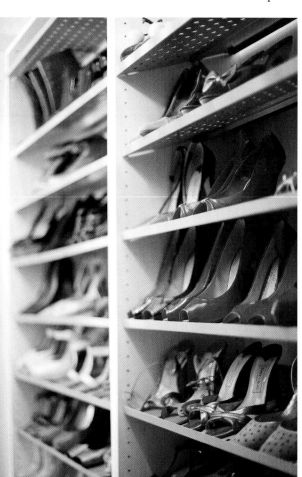

heels are a nice compromise because they don't kill and they look great with jeans. My rule for shoes is if the shoe hurts don't wear it! Never let salespeople talk you into buying a shoe that's a half size too big or too small. You will be in pain, which is never worth it.

My shoe wardrobe musts are as follows: a nice black pump, a tan nude pump, a few pairs of flats, a great wedge, and different boots. I like my flats to make a statement, which is why I buy nice ones that are embellished, including metallic flats with adornments and even gold ones. A sleek red pump is also a great evening look because any black outfit needs that pop. Coach always has great boot options, and I have Chloé boots from two seasons ago that I still love.

Remember that shoes change with every season. Pointy toes are in . . . then it's round toes. That's why I believe it's better not to spend a fortune on shoes. I really do think Steve Madden and

ALDO are fashion-conscious, wallet-conscious, and a girl's best friend. But if you invest in the expensive shoes, they will never go out of style. (The key is not to be a shoe-aholic.) If you're going to splurge, I would invest in expensive evening shoes. I have gold, silver, and black strappy heels from Jimmy Choo that always work and will never go out of style.

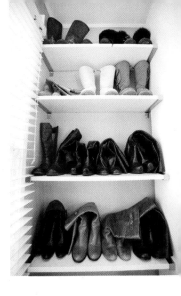

I have found Coach boots to not only be trendy but also timeless. I use them year after year. To me, that's worth the price. For super trendy shoes, go to Forever 21. Use them that year and guiltlessly throw them away when you've worn them out.

A Few Last Shoe Thoughts from Maria

- I always avoid wearing shoes with straps across the ankle. The strap cuts off the leg and makes me feel stubby. A sleek, sexy shoe that even has a little toe cleavage elongates the leg and works so much better.
- Avoid chunky heels. They look dated.
- Nude heels are my fave. Something shaped between a round toe and a pointed toe is perfect. And I love patent leather, too. ALDO has a nude pair now that I'm dying for because they go with everything and really help elongate the leg . . . unless you have darker skin. Then opt for a darker shoe.

Bathing Suits

Most women would rather have a root canal than try on new bathing suits. My advice is if you're going to try on a new bathing suit, then get a spray-tan. Realize that this will help, but no matter what, you will be miserable. I don't care how thin you are . . . it's never fun!

The problem is most suits have so much elastic in them that they squeeze you on the sides, and then you have the bulge. My best advice for bathing suits is to go a size bigger. Mine are eights on top and tens on the bottom. I have room, and I'm comfortable, and nothing is falling out.

You can't go wrong with the tankini, either. They're cute and they work, while hiding figure flaws. Also, be sure and get a cute cover-up dress and a plain cover-up. I have both and use them all the time.

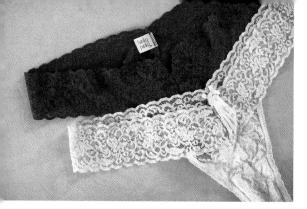

Hanky Panky makes the most comfortable thongs, and they come in gorgeous styles and colors. Victoria's Secret makes similar pairs for a lower budget.

Underwear

The main thing to remember with regard to underwear is *no granny panties, ever!* What you wear underneath your clothes sets the tone not only for your outfit but also your attitude. No matter what your size is, sexy undergarments will help you exude confidence. On a practical note, you don't want panty lines or wedgies, either! Ladies—just think of the day when you'll pass out from heatstroke and a hot EMT comes to your rescue. Do you really want to be caught in polka-dot granny panties?

My favorite underwear are thongs or G-strings. It all depends on what I'm wearing. Sometimes a G-string is cleaner under something that's tighter. My favorite brand of thong is Hanky Panky. Lace underwear is sexy to begin with, but these also wrap around your hips nicely, don't pull, and don't create any muffintop. Victoria's Secret recently created a knockoff line that's just as cool and a lot cheaper. I have both and the Hanky Pankys seem to last longer, but if you can't afford them, the Victoria's Secret line will do just fine!

What to Wear . . .

. . . To Your First Job Interview

Wearing a suit in a first interview is always a fine show of respect, but always take into consideration where you're interviewing. Some great accessories are nice, in addition to good hair and makeup. Be careful not to look dated. Do *not* wear the suit that's been in your closet for years or the suit that doesn't fit you right. It makes you look desperate and not up with the times. Never wear those old-style pin-striped suits. Throw them out. Look the part and you'll feel the part. Energy is contagious, so if you have a tired energy with a dated look, you will not get the part. Also, avoid anything too sexy or low cut, and wear an outfit that's clean and pressed. These seem obvious, but I've interviewed people who have erred on all of the above.

Maria's Three Interview Don'ts

1. DON'T wear shirts where your boobs are hanging out, for any job.
2. DON'T wear skirts so short that the person interviewing you is questioning whether you have underwear on.
3. DON'T wear ratty, stained, dirty, wrinkled, or outdated clothing.

. . . To Work

Dressing with style says so much about an employee. It says that you care about yourself and how you look while working. You represent the company well and show employers you have good taste and aptitude. You look like someone who has it together, and right out of the gate, it separates you from the pack.

Dress according to the environment you'll be working in. Office settings are generally conservative, and while that definitely doesn't condone hooker attire, it doesn't always mean suit, either. You can wear great slacks and a blouse with a belt and heels, as well as great accessories. Banana Republic has great Jackie O–style dresses to the knee, with skinny belts or just plain; add a scarf or great necklace. Voilà.

If you are going to work in a more laid-back atmosphere, wear something a little more trendy yet classy. I love a blazer, blouse, and jeans tucked into boots or with just a great pair of heels. A sweater-dress that's formfitting with leggings and heels, or a long cardigan over a T-shirt with a cute skirt accented with a waist belt are both fun outfits with conservative twists. You want to look modern and up with the times. Remember the movie *The Devil Wears Prada* and how Anne Hathaway's character dressed when her character was frumpy and not hip? That's *not* what *you* want to look like—especially when going into a hip environment. If you don't have hip clothes, or don't know where to start, head to H&M, Express, or even Forever 21, like I did. Among these stores, you can find a great outfit with cheap accessories that will make you look like you stepped out of a magazine. Print your favorite looks and head to the store and ask a sales clerk to help you find pieces to each look. It makes the process much faster and easier.

"Organize by outfit: this system works when you don't have oodles of time to decide on what to wear. Having a few tried-and-true looks you love hung together in your closet makes for easy-peasy access without too much effort."

—Stacy London, cohost of TLC's What Not to Wear *and cofounder of Style for Hire*

. . . On a First Date

My biggest tip for a first date is to not overdo it. Wear something casual with a splash of color. Color shows that you're fun. Jeans, a cute top, boots or heels, and an optional blazer are a perfect first-date look. You can't go wrong with the big three: jeans, boots, blazer. If it's a fancier date, then you can go for the LBD. It's much easier to have a daytime first date, when you can even do jeans, a baseball cap, a cute tee, and a little leather jacket.

. . . When You Have to Meet His Family

Don't be nervous. Just tone it down with the clothes and go back to your first-date look. You want to look relatable to his mother and father. Remember that first impressions are lasting and his parents want to be proud of the girl their son is bringing home. This is never the time to wear a low-cut top. Think of this like a job interview. Do a pop of color to show your warm side.

AND MY NOT-SO-JUICY RULE

If you are thirty-something or more, do not wear hypercolored Juicy sweat suits. It's cheesy. Walking around LA, I see women in bright lime-green or hot-pink sweat outfits, which also come in horrifying bright yellow. Sweats were a big fad. We wore them all the time for all occasions. Today's style is to wear them less—just for lounging around or working out.

. . . For the Romantic Weekend Getaway

Pack as lightly as possible. You never want to be the girl who shows up with ten suitcases for two days. Pack one pair of jeans, your bathing suit, something to sleep in (or not), two great T-shirts, and maybe your LBD and a blazer. Wear flats and the bulkier items on the plane and pack your lingerie and heels. Workout clothes are optional. Bring three to four accessories to shake it up a bit. Resolve that you will wear your white T-shirt under your blazer the first night, and the next day under a cardigan.

. . . Going from Day to Night

The other day, I was at *Access Hollywood* and knew that I had to go to both day and night events. So during the day I wore leggings with flats and a long pink top that covered my butt. Later, I added a blazer and a fun long necklace, plus my Stuart Weitzman over-the-knee boots. It was a cute outfit for both day and night; plus, the leggings were comfortable and sexy.

If you can wear jeans to work, then bring a great leather bomber jacket and tank for night. Add some amazing jewelry and boots or heels. Or add red heels to make the outfit pop (they look great with jeans). A white tank, black leather jacket, jeans, and red heels is a great day-to-night look. If you wear a sleeveless dress, then throw a leather jacket on top of it to go from day to night.

> **EveryGirl Extra-Credit Tip:** If your BFF lives far away, use Skype to see if she likes your outfit.

> **EveryGirl Extra-Credit Tip:** Keep the extra buttons from all your new clothing in one place.

> **EveryGirl Extra-Credit Tip:** Clothes-swap with friends. It's a fun and recession-happy event.

While You're at It, Dress Up Your Mom

She dressed you as a girl, and now it might be your turn to give her wardrobe a little light makeover. The problem with most moms is they have a vast collection of clothing they don't wear anymore jamming their closets. The first step here is (if you can) having a closet-cleaning day with Mom. I did this with my mom and took her on a little shopping spree, where we bought nice slacks and great tops at New York & Company. I didn't get her separates because half the time she wouldn't remember how to pull them together. When we went in there, I said, "I need five really strong outfits for my mom." We bought mostly solids and even took pictures on my phone so Mom could remember exactly how the outfits went together. By the way, Mom wore her twenty-dollar camisole under a blazer with gorgeous slacks to my birthday party a week later and looked absolutely gorgeous.

A Maria Fashionista Moment (or Two or Three!)

I interview celebs about fashion on a daily basis. Here are a few of my favorite stories from the fashion front lines.

- Ever show up at a wedding wearing the same dress as another guest? Two years ago, in Cannes, at a private dinner for Valentino thrown by Chopard, Minnie Driver and I showed up in the same white Valentino dress. All you can do is laugh it off.
- I picked a dress to wear for the 2010 Oscars. While watching the Grammys, I saw Pink walk in . . . in the dress I had hoped to wear a month later. Oh well, we both have great taste!
- At the 2009 Video Music Awards, Pink and Shakira walked the red carpet wearing the same dress. I broke the news to Shakira. She whipped around and found Pink in the same dress, and they posed for pictures together. Both ladies were totally cool about it.
- My strangest fashion experience happened at the Playboy Mansion. I was there to interview the Kardashians. Looking around for them, I walked around a corner and saw naked women who had "clothes" painted on them. It was just so bizarre because they wanted to take pictures with me. I had no idea what to do with my hands!
- At a 2009 Burberry event, I wore a great Burberry outfit with a gorgeous necklace that just killed me. This thing weighed about a thousand pounds and was crafted with heavy daggerlike metal pieces. I was in actual pain. Finally, I had the waiter wrap a cloth napkin around the back of the necklace so it stayed off my skin. By the way, I had a bruise for quite some time. The red carpet shot hit all of the magazines and my outfit was a hit! In fashion, as in life: no pain, no gain.

Your Wardrobe Fix-It Kit

Have these at hand at all times:

- Double-sided tape for your boobs, a hemline that rips, and everything in between
- Dryer sheets for static cling
- Tide to Go Instant Stain Remover for stains
- Baby wipes for deodorant marks
- Little scissors
- Pins

EveryGirl Extra-Credit Tip: Beware of see-through dresses. I wore one once, and you could see my pasties through the dress. For me, what's horrifying is that there is a red carpet snap of this out there! The best way to judge is to take a picture of yourself in the light. The camera will be your mortification guide and will pick up what you can't. (The pic ended up in *Playboy*, by the way!)

I wore this beautiful custom-made Ralph & Russo dress to the Emmys. It made me feel so glamorous.

And the sexy design of the back highlighted my curves. Choose clothes to accentuate your best assets.

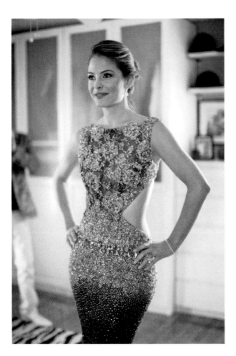

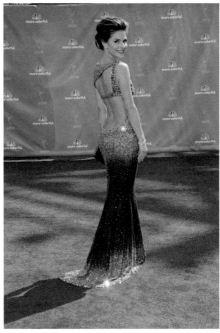

EveryGirl Hair and Nails

A Pantene EveryGirl

When I was growing up, my *theia* Anna (that's "aunt" in Greek) always cut my hair. She still owns and operates a salon in Everett, Massachusetts, called Sebastian's. *Thanks for all the free hair cuts, Theia!* And believe it or not, Pantene was always a staple in my house. At fifteen, the Barbizon Modeling School would send me to CVS stores all over the state to educate consumers on the shampoo! I had trifold boards with information on Pro-V, and samples to boot, and would teach customers about

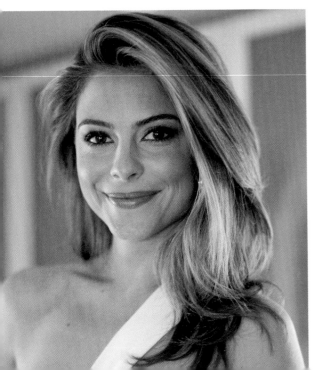

it. Coincidentally, ten years later I became *the* Pantene spokesmodel. When the executives at Pantene told me I got the gig, I said, "Wow, I've been working for you guys since I was fifteen!" I told them the story, and I think at that point they knew they had the right girl for the job. I truly believe in the product and can honestly say it's what I've used for my entire life.

The toughest part of shooting the commercials was actually getting my hair color straight. Colorist Patti Song and I would spend an entire day coloring my hair for each shoot, and we've become great friends as a result.

On set, you'd be surprised to hear that styl-

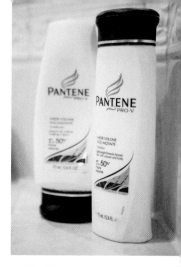

ing my hair was the *easiest* part of the process. The stylist, Serena, would put my hair in Velcro rollers and leave them in during makeup. Two hours later, when she'd take my hair out of the rollers, it would be huge! Using the Volumizing Collection with the Velcro rollers really did make my hair that enormous. I thought for sure they would ask me to wear false hair or something. Seeing girls in the commercials before me, I figured there was no way that hair could get that full unless it was fake. But great product and technique actually do the trick.

Even though we spend so much money having our hair professionally fixed and so many hours fussing with it, to have gorgeous hair you really don't have to spend a fortune. I don't have as much training in hair care as I do in makeup. However, between my experiences with Team Pantene and the fact that I work with the world's best stylists, I've learned enough to do my own hair for events and TV and in the usual time- and cost-effective ways. I'm always excited when I land in a magazine and can say, "I did that look myself!"

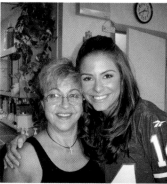

My aunt Anna and me at her hair salon.

Taking Care of Your Hair

Shampoo and Condition

I don't shell out a lot of cash on shampoo or conditioner because it's absolutely unnecessary. I know we live in an age where designer shampoos can be expensive, but women do not need to spend that much. I have known friends who break the bank to buy shampoo and conditioner and wouldn't even consider anything else. If you are rich and can afford the finer things in life, by all means do so, but debt over these items is not smart.

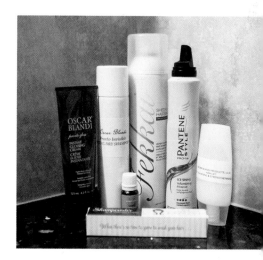

Perhaps you've heard that your hair gets used to a certain shampoo or conditioner, and then it doesn't work as effectively over time. Guess what? That's true. Long-term use of any product creates buildup from that exact mix. That's why I have different products in the shower and even try new products every now and then. Ladies with natural hair colors can also try a clarifying rinse of apple cider vinegar to get rid of buildup. And how do you know if you have buildup? Your hair stops responding to your favorite products and looks dull and lifeless. The main shampoo and conditioners in my shower right now are from Pantene Pro-V's Volumizing Collection and Pantene Pro-V's Brunette Expressions. My favorite splurge shampoo is Frédéric Fekkai Brilliant Glossing Shampoo. It's a shine-enhancing, color-protecting cleanser, meaning it is safe for color-treated hair.

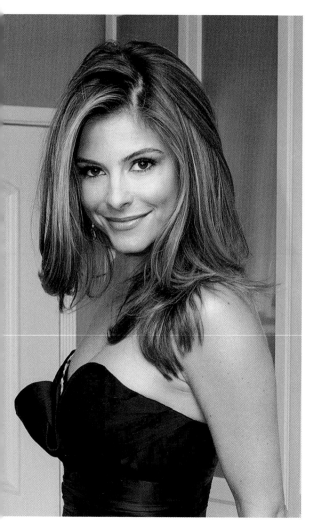

How to Get Maximum Shine

There's nothing more glam and gorgeous than healthy-looking hair that has a natural shine. Clean hair rinsed in cold water should be shiny. Shine serums, sprays, and glossing creams can help achieve this look, too. Oscar Blandi makes an amazing product called Pronto Gloss Instant Glossing Cream. I put it on my towel-dried hair, and it is so lightweight you don't even know it's there. If you can't afford that, Clairol Jazzing is another affordable product Patti taught me about. It's a clear gloss treatment you put on your hair in the shower like a mask and rinse. The results last a long time. Or you can try Pantene Fine Hair Heat Protection & Shine Spray. I love my two-in-one products! The spray protects your hair from styling damage and gives it great shine at the same time.

Give Your Hair a Break

Many of us color our hair and then jump into a daily routine of blow-drying combined with a curling iron or hair-straightening device. This can really damage your hair. If your locks feel dry and look like straw, your hair is begging for a break. Stop doing all of the above and give your hair a rest. Use the heated styling tools only when you're going out or need to look great, which isn't daily. Or give your hair a break on the weekends. Having an attached diffuser on your blow-dryer will minimize damaging effects, as well. When my hair gets really damaged, I air-dry it and am always cautious, using a heat protectant before applying any heat.

MARIA HAIR REMEDIES

- Clip split ends. I will sit forever and carefully cut mine. Doing so makes the hair grow out healthily. Just remember to never cut more than the split end, as you want to avoid hair becoming different lengths.
- Get trims every six weeks to keep it healthy.
- Choose simple hairdos that don't require any teasing or too much product when hair is damaged. Also try to let it air-dry as often as possible.
- Be careful not to rip elastics out of hair, and be super gentle with it.
- Regular hair masks can revive hair from the dead.
- Use color (highlights or full color) every two to three months rather than every six to eight weeks. That's an easy way to reduce split ends and keep your shine on. Plus, you'll be saving money and will still look good. Sarah Jessica Parker shows a little hint of roots and looks gorgeous.
- Towel-dry when possible.
- Try Jessica Simpson's HairDo extensions. Pop a piece in and your hair instantly looks great—no styling necessary. Now you can really give your hair the break it needs!
- Make sure to always wash out your conditioner with cool water to lock in all of its benefits. Remember that cool water seals your hair cuticles and makes your hair shiny. Hot water sucks the moisture right out of your scalp. I shower with hot water but change to cool water when I wash my hair.

Vitamins, Supplements, and Foods for Healthy Hair

Many of the vitamins and foods you need to consume for good skin are equally beneficial for hair and even nails. Here is a list:

- A whole-food multivitamin
- Vitamins A, C, E, and B complex (also helps keep gray hairs away)
- Biotin
- Niacin
- Silica
- Plenty of greens, raw seeds and nuts, avocados, citrus fruits, bell peppers, cold-water fish, brown rice, soybeans (tofu is great), red grapes, tomatoes, and cold-pressed oils
- Three to five liters of purified water daily

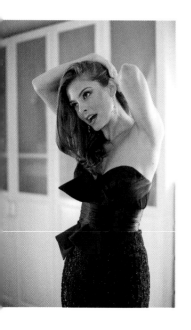

RUB YOUR HEAD

Jon Bon Jovi is a star who rocks the most gorgeous mane of hair. Ask him his secret and he will admit that he has done a daily scalp massage on himself since he was in his twenties. It's a great idea that top hairdressers recommend to their clients. Gently rub the pads of your fingertips on your scalp in circular motions for about five minutes a day. You can also do this during your shampooing. Good hair health starts with a healthy scalp. A light massage not only feels good but also brings more blood to your scalp area, which promotes healthy hair growth.

Getting Cut

I know many women are cutting back on haircuts in order to save money. It's a smart idea to save money in any way possible, but you don't want to mess your hair up, either. Longer hair requires less maintenance and less money than short hair, so consider keeping your hair long and find a cheaper place to do your trims every six to eight weeks. A trim is often much less expensive than a major cut. And that trim really does help keep away split ends, which will make your hair look worn-out and tired.

A cheaper place may have less talented stylists (I say "may" because I've met many diamonds in the rough over the years), but it's just a trim, not a full cut. They'll be less likely to mess up.

Long Hair Isn't Just for Teenagers!

One of the things I find most disheartening is the fact that women think they can't have long hair after a certain age. Jaclyn Smith, Cheryl Ladd, Lauren Hutton, Janice Dickinson, Suzanne Somers, and a long list of other women rock long hair into their sixties, and so should everyone else if long hair looks good on them. My mom recently let her hair grow out. Now when we look at pictures of her from ten years ago and compare them to today, we think she looks twenty years younger with her longer locks.

Getting the Right Cut

I love my hairstylist Olivier Geymann, stylist at Serge Normant at John Frieda Salaon in Los Angeles. Olivier cuts my hair and many other famous manes, including Charlize Theron's and Dana Delany's. Here are Olivier's best hair tips for the EveryGirl.

Face Shape

A round-shaped face is as wide as it is long, with soft, round edges. AVOID short curly hair, short cropped styles, and styles that add volume at the sides.

An oval-shaped face has a length that is equal to one and a half times the width. AVOID short layers that add height to the crown or top of the head, and blunt cuts if the hair is too curly or thick.

A rectangular-shaped face is long, with a more angular appearance. AVOID long hair; this will make the face look longer. Also avoid super-short styles.

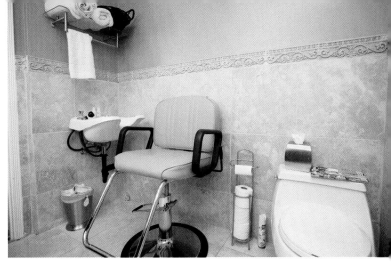

Because my job requires me to always have my hair done, I set up a mini hair salon counter in my spare bathroom. It was an investment that has been well worth the time I save.

A square-shaped face is as wide as it is long but with more of an angular appearance, rather than a round appearance.
AVOID chin-length bobs and blunt bangs.
A heart-shaped face has a narrow jaw and is wider at the forehead or cheekbones, or both.
AVOID choppy layers, super-short hair, and volume at the crown.

FOR THINNING HAIR

DermMatch is a makeup-style powder (applied much like a compact) that is rubbed on to thinning areas with a brush. DermMatch comes in all hair colors and remains on when swimming, perspiring, or in the rain; it only comes off after shampooing. Sold online, DermMatch is less than thirty dollars.

"Don't fight a bad hair day! I always think a ponytail is the way to go. You can go for a high or low one depending on your mood. Always have bobby pins or an elastic band or headband on you."

—Melanie Mezzacappa, celebrity hairstylist

MARIA'S DOS AND DON'TS OF GREAT HAIR

- DO get trims every six to eight weeks.
- It's not cute or attractive to be a greaseball. Use Shampowder by Buttercream Cosmetics to soak up grease.
- DO comb your hair. As you comb through your hair, it helps spread the *natural* oils. Start from the bottom and work your way up to protect your hair.
- DO apply sunblock to the hair and scalp.
- DON'T go overboard with your highlights. A kiss of color is the way to go.
- DO use Pantene mousse. It's a hairdresser fave, as well as mine.
- DON'T wash your hair every day. I wash mine twice a week.

Red Carpet Hair

These are some of my favorite red carpet hair looks:

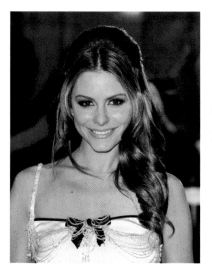

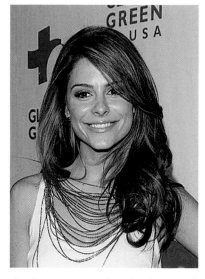

This look is great for a first date or your friend's wedding: Half up/half down with a twist. I wore my hair like this for the Benjamin Button premiere. Before putting half of your hair in a ponytail, tease the top. Then split some bangs down either side in the front and use a big curling iron to achieve the curl.

On the green carpet here for the annual Global Green event. P.S. My dress was made from 100 percent milk! I was truly green! To get the look on your hair, use a big curling iron and only curl halfway to your scalp. I like this as a great everyday look that easily blends to night.

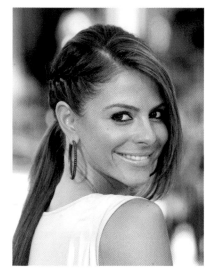

A ponytail with an edge! Yet another Brad Pitt premiere, this time for Inglourious Basterds. Braid one side of your hair and tie with a small ponytail holder. Minus a side-swept clump of bangs, use all of your hair, including the mini braid, and make another ponytail. Wrap the ponytail with some of your hair for a clean finished look. If you're headed to a concert or any kind of fun event, this will set you apart from the crowd.

"One basic hair-styling tip. If you want to add volume to flat hair, try twisting it up in a high bun in the morning on your commute. When you let it down, the bun will have created a natural wave."

—Tommy Cyr, celebrity hairstylist

EveryGirl Extra-Credit Tip: If you can't afford a pricey salon, then have your hair cut at a local hair school. The price will be cheaper, and you can ask for a more advanced student.

EveryGirl Extra-Credit Tip: The biggest fader of colored hair is the sun, so use a sunscreen for your hair when going outdoors. Try Frédéric Fekkai's Marine Summer Hair Beachcomber Leave-in Conditioner. If you are going to be at the beach, wear a silk scarf or floppy hat.

EveryGirl Extra-Credit Tip: In between appointments, when you see roots but can't get in for an appointment, you can try color pens to fill in roots. I use Osar Blandi Pronto Colore.

COLOR BY KYLE

Celebrity colorist Kyle White of the Oscar Blandi Salon in New York, colors my hair. Here is his expert advice on coloring your hair.

Choosing the right color:

Kyle says that your hair color should balance out or be the opposite of your skin tone. If you have a "warm" skin tone (with pink or red undertones, like Renée Zellweger or other fair-skinned beauties), you need a "cool" hair color like platinum, baby blonde, or sandy and beige blondes, NOT the warm golden blondes and strawberry blonde, which have hints of red in them. If you have a "cool" skin tone (with green/olive and yellow undertones, like Sophia Loren), you need a warm hair color like a chestnut brown, golden brown, or even a dark red, *not* coffee or sandy brown. Simply put, warm hair color dyes contain hints of red or gold, and cool hair color dyes contain no red or gold.

Finding a great colorist who will pick out the best shade for your complexion is priceless, so don't forget to tip your colorist. Kyle recommends 15 to 20 percent of the cost.

Once you've colored your hair, protect it with a deep-conditioning treatment once a week. Kyle recommends using a leave-in protein spray every time you wash, and not shampooing every day of the week.

Gorgeous Hands and Nails

There's nothing more beautiful than gorgeous hands, but often this is an overlooked area for many busy women. We all invest so much money on our faces and forget areas like our hands. The good news is it's easy and takes very little time to keep your hands and nails in great shape. Use these tips to make sure that your hands look lovely at all times.

- Remember to put sunscreen on the backs of your hands. Many stars keep a bottle of sunscreen in their cars to make sure that their hands get a little extra protection while driving. Sun will quickly age your hands.

- You can use a bit of your face serum and moisturizer on your hands to keep the skin younger-looking and line-free. Your hands will quickly respond to retinols, peptides, and alpha-hydroxy acids. I always use excess face products I've used on my skin, like moisturizers and serums, on my hands.

Nails

Clean, manicured nails are a must. However, maintaining them can take a lot of time and money. It certainly does for me. Like all things, I've found some shortcuts around it all. Let's go over some options.

Acrylic Nails

Acrylic nails have been around for a long time. I got acrylic nails when I first moved to LA. They need to be redone every two to three weeks. I quickly grew tired of the upkeep and went au naturel.

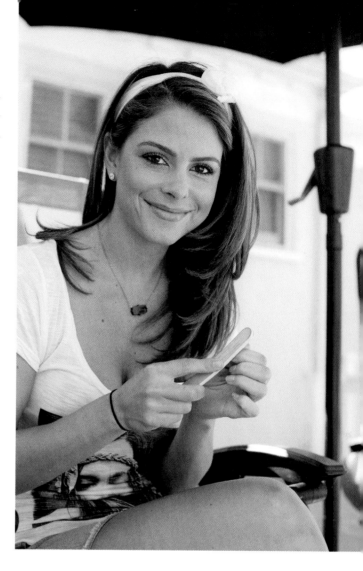

Gel Nails

Gel nails are a newer artificial nail that many women prefer over acrylic because of their flexibility, which makes them less prone to cracks and chips. They are faster to apply, not as thick, and more natural-looking than acrylics, too. Also, gel nails are odorless and don't require the strong-smelling chemicals to apply or remove them, like acrylic nails do. Curing time for gel nails is shorter than for the acrylic ones. They do come at a price, though!

To be honest, I don't recommend either type of nail—unless you just have really unhealthy or super-weak nails (then I'd say get gel nails).

EveryGirl Extra-Credit Tip: Be sure and purchase the nail polish you use most. You can get more mileage out of your mani/pedi if you have the polish to touch up.

One reason I opt against them is because both processes are damaging to your real nails. Gel nails aren't as severe, but they are still damaging when removed. The other big reasons are the time and money. For me, it's just one more thing to do during my packed day. Instead, I keep my nails short and buff them instead of polishing. You can buy a buffer at any drugstore. Buff your nails with rapid movements, as if you're filing the top of your nails, until they're shiny.

Pedicure

As much as you want to save time and money, you do not want to have gross-looking toenails. When I had to make budget cuts, I decided manicures I could do without; pedicures were just too important. I make sure to have the pedicurist cut my toenails short, making the need for visits a bit less frequent. Another way I maintain my pedicure for almost a month is by filing the nails as they get longer. I do this carefully so as not to chip the polish, and it works like a charm. I end up spending less than twenty dollars per month on my nails, and that works great for me!

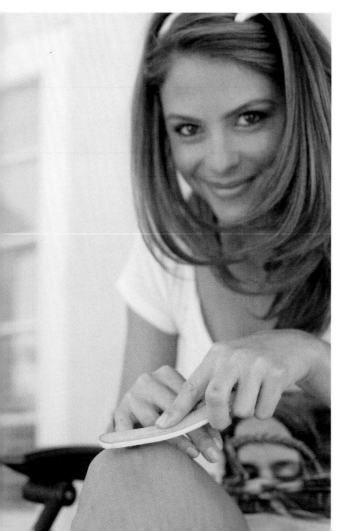

Buffing nails is a cheap and easy way to make your nails look great!

A Few Other Nail Tricks

- If you've used dark polish that has stained your nails, wipe whitening toothpaste on your nail beds. The stain will vanish.
- Use fresh pineapple to push back your cuticles naturally. Just rub it on your fingertips and then push back your cuticles. The acid in the pineapple will help you get rid of any jagged cuticles.
- Clean underneath your fingernails using a wet cotton swab for long nails and a cuticle pusher wrapped in tissue for short nails. They carry bacteria and germs beneath them.

EveryGirl Extra-Credit Tip: Kim, the manicurist at my local salon, taught me how to keep a manicure for two weeks. It sounds impossible, but I tried it and it worked. After you get your nails done, do not do anything strenuous with your hands for twenty-four hours. I know it's hard, but if you guard them, it works. Even if you shower the next morning, be gentle with them when washing your hair. The goal is to protect the tip and if you do, you'll be thanking me two weeks later! Remember: no digging in the purse!

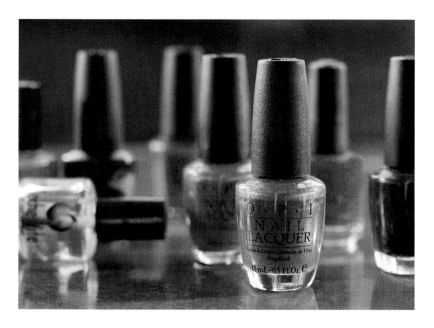

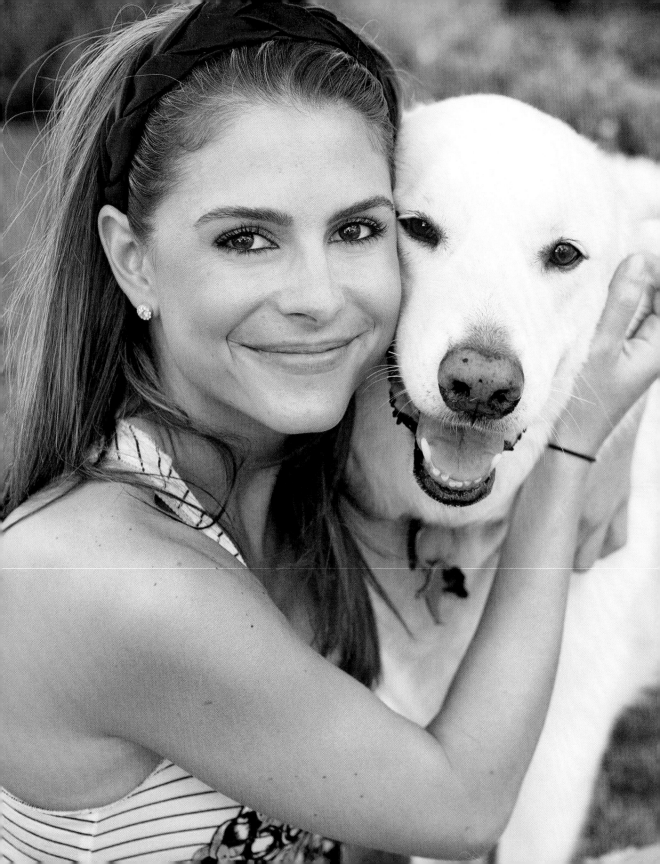

part three

EveryGirl Emotional Foundation

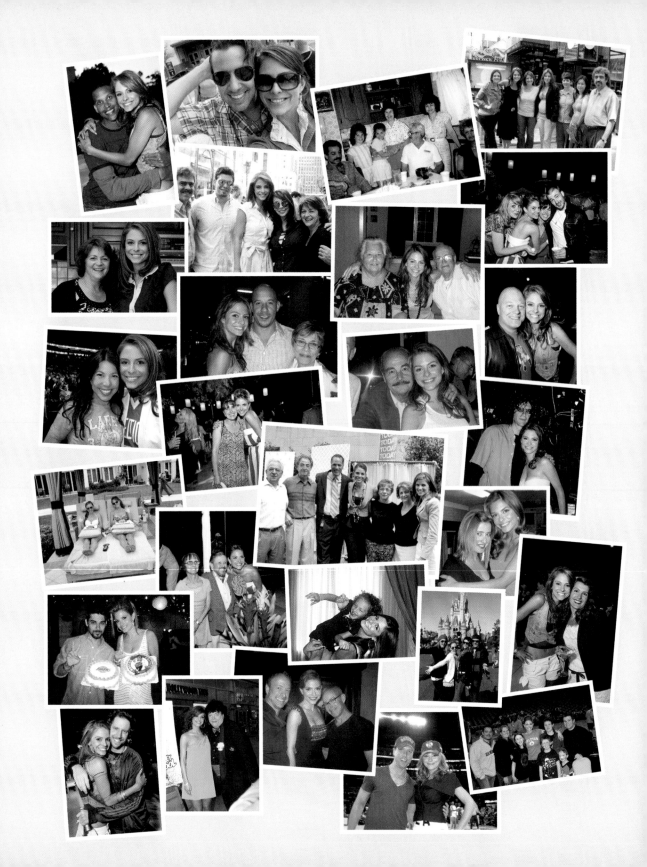

So what exactly defines a strong emotional foundation? It's one layered with high self-esteem and self-confidence, as well as the presence of friends, family, and partners who love and support you unconditionally. Having this kind of friend and family is a crucial part of your foundation. Conversely, the wrong kind of friends and family will erode, and even destroy, your foundation.

My goal is to help you to choose and to nurture the right ones while avoiding and distancing yourself from the wrong ones.

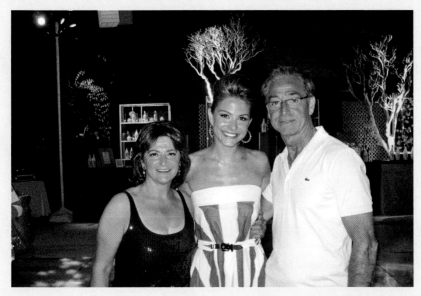

My parents and me at my thirtieth birthday party at my home in Los Angeles.

CHAPTER NINE

EveryGirl Friends and Family

There are times in your life that literally change you to the core. For me, this time was during college, beginning when I volunteered to work on the film *In the Land of Merry Misfits*. This is how I met Keven. It was his film and he worked with an eclectic bunch of non-Hollywood types, to say the least. Many would become my new friends and positively impact my life.

Seek Diversity in Friendships

Now let me tell you the official statuses of these people when I met them. They were: an apartment manager, a caretaker, a coffee shop clerk, a hospital attendant, a shopkeeper, a travel agent, a construction worker, and a carny. They were not big-time movers and shakers. They were not the "cool" friends that most people are attracted to. But they were generous, kind, and unique human beings who wanted good things for me. Those are the true qualities we should all seek in friends. Good things sprouted in my life as a result of my friendships with them.

I had high school friends and family frown on me for participating in these friendships, since they were open to relationships only with people from similar backgrounds.

Thank God, I didn't care what everyone else

Here I am with my In the Land of Merry Misfits *cast.*

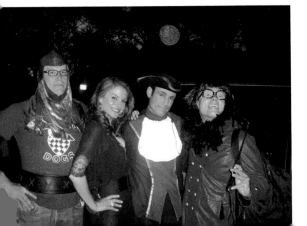

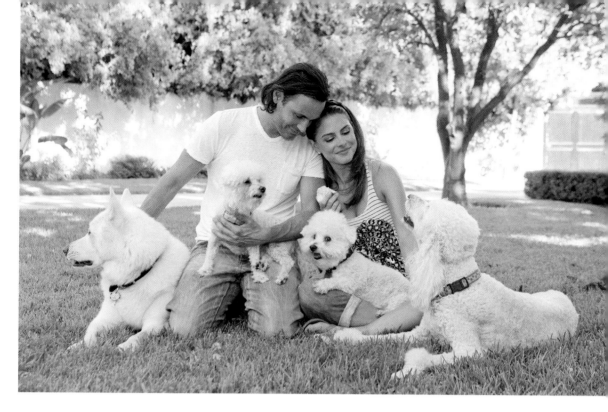

thought. I went to kindergarten not knowing one word of English and speaking only Greek. Nia Vardalos's *My Big Fat Greek Wedding* captured the loneliness of what a lot of us Greek kids experienced, and probably what kids from most first-generation immigrant families or different social classes experience, for that matter. I think this made me more sensitive to others who are different and forced me to be open to all kinds of friendships, too. Be sure to do the same.

EveryGirl Motto:
Seek diversity in your friendships. It's far more enriching. Closing off from it stunts your growth.

A Good Friend

A good friend, to me, is:

- Someone who is there for you when you need him or her.
- Someone who is a good listener.
- Someone who will defend you in tough times, and yet has the courage to stand up to you and be honest.
- Someone who inspires you and helps make you a better person.
- Someone who wants to see you succeed.
- Someone who is respectful.

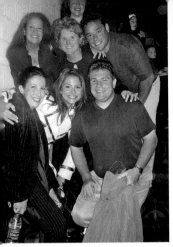

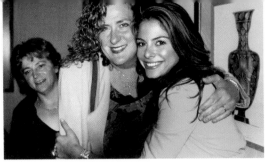

I always called Sophia Carafotes my "Big Sis" and I still do! We met at church.

I took my family to the movies to see my film debut in the Fantastic Four.

PLACES TO MEET NEW FRIENDS

- Volunteer for a charity. It is a great, fast way to meet friends who have similar concerns and ideals. Check out groups you would like to support on the Internet.
- Stick around after church, temple, or synagogue services and talk to people. You can also join their social groups.
- Explore hobbies to meet new people. Love scuba diving? Join a local group. Want to paint? Take art lessons.

FRIENDLY ACTIVITIES

Book clubs, knitting clubs, and cooking clubs continue to be popular. There's no reason you can't be part of any of them or create innovative clubs of your own. Why don't you . . .

- Organize a weekly game of your favorite sport? I have a weekly Sunday hoops game each spring.
- Create an unofficial club with friends to watch your favorite TV shows for a fun laugh? (I knew of a *Rock of Love* club.) We started AfterBuzz TV, a podcast where we break down episodes from our favorite TV scenes, as an excuse to get together with friends. Once a week, friends and I will watch TV together, then gab about it. It's so much fun.
- Organize clothing swaps with your friends, where everyone brings clothes they are throwing out? Draw straws to determine who picks first and in what order, and then swap. It's green, it's free, and it's fun!
- Go hiking with girlfriends? It's great exercise and a way for you and your GFs to vent and decompress about your weeks. Or split a trainer session. I do this with my friend Rachel as a way to get together.
- Pitch in with the gals to hire a masseur to come over for the day at a reduced rate? Normally a masseur might charge $125 an hour, or $575 for five of you. Instead, offer $300. Even $60 an hour is nothing to sneeze at—especially in this economy.

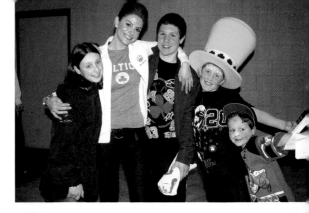

The Sparages clan and me at the Celtics game. I love my little cousins!

If Possible—Stay Close with Old Friends

So, does meeting new friends mean you need to ditch your old friends? Absolutely not! Alyssa Wallerce has been my best friend since I was in eighth grade. On the occasions I can get home to Boston, I'll often forgo nights at the Ritz-Carlton on the company dime just to have sleepovers with her family. Alyssa always tells it to me straight, and everyone needs that type of friend.

Alyssa knows me so well and has been there for me in tough moments. A few years ago while at the Cannes Film Festival, I got very ill. I contracted some rare intestinal infection and spent the week in a French hospital. To make matters worse, after flying home, I learned that my grandmother had passed away. I needed to go home and be with my mom but I was so weak I couldn't make the flight alone. Alyssa, who works for United, flew to the West Coast and thirty minutes after she landed, she flew right back to Boston with me. Now, *that's* a friend. To this day I can always call on her.

The Carafotes sisters remain the older sisters I never had. We sang in church choir together from the time I was twelve. As teachers, they even helped me with my pageants, instructing me about public speaking. They have always supported and loved me unconditionally.

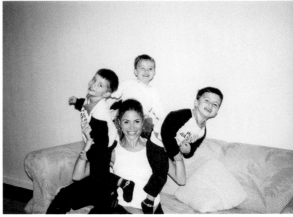

Here I am with my godson, Kimon; Iraklis; and Othon.

Old friends keep you true to your roots and provide a unique familiarity and comfort. Just don't let that comfortable feeling close you off from meeting new friends, because you have enough room in your life to mix the old with the new here.

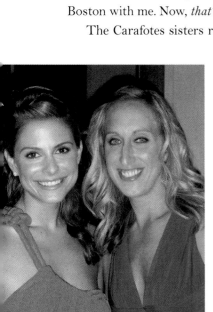

Alyssa and me pictured here at an event I hosted. I gave her this dress that I wore in a Pantene Commercial

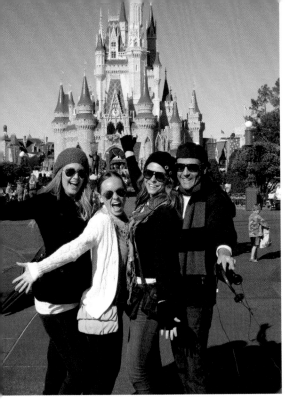

Valerie, Cate, Keven, and me at Disney World.

Young or Old

Another tip I live by is the one I got from Ron Piretti, one of my friends and a star from *Misfits*. Ron, who's in his seventies, told me that when you get old, you should hang out with young people. Ron is an energetic guy whose mind is always "in possibility." He was frustrated with people his own age who were just content spending their remaining years tired, bored, negative, and in a constant state of complaint. He felt those people were just waiting to die. Young people still have dreams. They inspire him and help him continue to grow. All things considered, it's always healthy to have friends younger than you. It doesn't hurt to be a mentor to them, either.

The reverse of Ron's rule applies, too. When you're young, hang out with old people. Older people have wisdom and life experience that young people don't. I have always reached out to older people and do so to this very day. The majority of my close friends are at least ten years older than me. They've "lived it," and their advice is invaluable, as is their friendship.

How do you find older people and younger people to become friends with? It's the same as finding new friends. Work is always a great source, but don't rule out places like old-age homes or youth centers, where you can volunteer. Again, it's really a matter of being open to the prospect, while living your life, that will yield results.

The Sunshine Committee

My friend Randal Malone, also from *Misfits*, donates his time to working with the elderly, and one of his char-

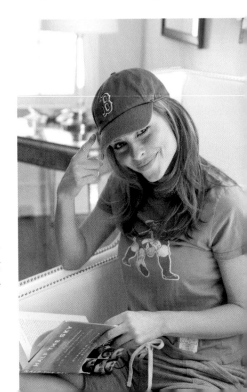

Staying true to my Boston roots.

ity groups has a committee called the Sunshine Committee. The women on this committee make table settings, order flowers, and arrange for entertainment. The name stuck with me, and for years it's become my name for people in life who actually bring the sunshine. These are the people who are positive, happy, and believe in possibility. I try to surround myself only with people from the Sunshine Committee.

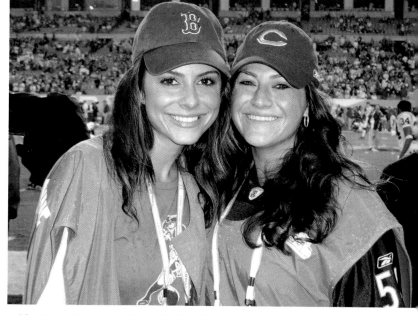

My former assistant and now BFF Meredith Ahern with me at a football game.

The EveryGirl Advisory Committee

Any company CEO has an advisory committee to bounce ideas off and solicit assistance from, and a CEO like you shouldn't be any different. My committee consists of friends and family, many of whom I've already mentioned in the book. These are people I go to for answers to questions about my career, my relationships, and my life in general.

You may already have a support committee in your life, too, but if you don't, then create one. This committee doesn't have to meet like other committees do, and its members don't even need to know one another. They need only to be people in your life who will give you sound, honest advice and unconditional love. These are the people you go to when you need answers—especially important ones. They will help you make the big decisions. Remember that you hold veto power and the final say. As always, be certain to offer the same support to these friends in return.

EveryGirl Motto: Make sure your friends are people who root for you. Are they on "Team You"? Make this a prerequisite for all friendships. It goes both ways. You need to root for the success of your friends just like they root for you.

EveryGirl Friends . . . to Lose

There are "friends" who you cannot keep and "friends" you should make every effort to avoid. These are the ones who are jealous of you and the

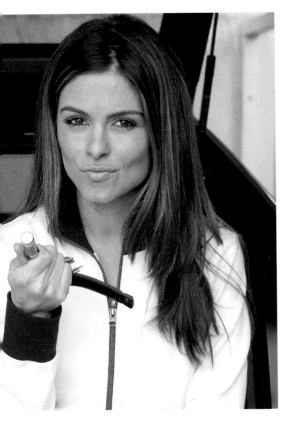

For the record, I'm holding a lipstick can of pepper spray. I keep mine attached to my key ring at all times. I have it out and ready in parking lots. I've known too many girls who've been mugged or held at gunpoint. Be safe!

ones who secretly do not root for your success. Or they're negative or just a bad influence. Any of the above will erode your foundation for sure. These are the friends to lose.

I know it isn't easy. Many bad friends whom we've known forever fit into a comfort zone, and it's hard to step away. You just have to do it. They are bags of bricks—and not the kind used to build strong foundations—the kind you just lug around and exhaust yourself carrying, the kind that serve no purpose other than to drain or, worse, hurt you.

Avoid Vampires

As hot as the guys from *Twilight* are, you need to avoid real-life vampires. Who are the real-life vampires? They're people who suck your energy or destroy you. Vampires come in many varieties, and I've known many. Vampire Paul was trying to steal props off my movie set. Vampire Karen is a coworker who complains about work and life every minute of the day. Vampire Dan talks only about himself and demands every minute of my time. I'm sure you know many vampires, too. Do your best to distance yourself from them.

What Kind of Friend Are They to Others?

Are your friends there in the bad times? Do they gossip about other friends to you or others you know? When they feel they've been wronged, do they respond in a healthy manner, by speaking up in a civilized tone or even walking away with class? Or do they throw a brick through the other party's window, key their cars, or attack them physically? (I'm a city girl and, unfortunately, I've seen "friends" do this.)

If you notice people acting or reacting in this manner, then distance yourself from them. They may not have done anything to you yet, but if you happen to stumble into their crosshairs, chances are good that they will turn on you, too.

Dr. Gail's Advice for the EveryGirl

Dr. Gail Saltz is a top psychiatrist and psychoanalyst, columnist, and best-selling author who specializes in relationship issues. She has appeared on *The Oprah Winfrey Show* and is one of my friends from the *Today* show. She was kind enough to talk to EveryGirls out there about issues revolving around friendships and family.

Q: What do you do if a friendship is clearly becoming one-sided? It's all about their schedule and their needs . . . their boyfriend, their problems, their plans. Should you opt out of that relationship?

A: First, you need to realize that there are many different kinds of friendships and not all friends are created equal. Sadly, we've gotten to a point with Facebook that you have to ask yourself, "What is a friend?" You can have zillions of friends you don't even know. The bad news here is we've become cavalier about friendship. What you need to know is that not every friend has to be the most intense, perfect relationship. You don't need to always see eye to eye. And it doesn't always have to be a fair trade. The key with friends is you don't have to like everything about them, but you must like more things about them than you don't like.

Q: So what happens when it's not an equal exchange?

A: Both of you should mutually get something out of the relationship. The problem is sometimes a friendship gravitates toward one or the other person. You're no longer equal and the vector moves one way. You need to realize that friendships go through periods where she will get more—or you will get more. You can be in need and demand more from friends, and that's okay. I'm a big believer in valuing your relationships and being there for your friends. Remember that relationships are the most important thing you have in life and the biggest source of happiness. So give friends a chance even if there is a period where she gets much more. Don't just bolt out of the friendship.

Q: What if you do want to discuss a troubled friendship? What is a kind way to approach that discussion?

A: First, identify that there is trouble in the relationship. Tell your friend, "There's something wrong and I want to talk about it. I really value our friendship, but I notice . . ." Now, fill in the blanks. Finish by saying, "I really want to work on this with you. It's important to me to keep this relationship with you." The key is to keep the lines of communication wide open.

Q: When should you end a friendship?

A: Ask yourself if the other person is worth it to you. Are they capable of change? Will they put in the work to save the friendship? If they're not capable of change and won't work on it, then it might be time to leave. But I don't think you always have to have a big ending with a friendship. There are friendships where you just naturally drift away. You might come back to these friends at a later time in life.

Q: Okay, you met a guy and your girlfriends are jealous and mad at you. They're even talking badly about your new guy. What should you do?

A: It's so common for women to be very close friends and then one meets a guy. Suddenly, one party is not so close. They're investing more in the relationship with the man than the friendship. That's very normal behavior. Moderation is key here. Don't overreact. If you're the friend who has been ignored because your girlfriend has a new man, just say to her, "I really miss you. I know you're really into Ron and I'm so happy for you. I'm not trying to be your wife here, but I do miss the time we used to spend together. Maybe we could try to work out a few things to do together." But know the reality of life is that people have new relationships and they won't have enough time for you. The friend on the outside shouldn't be extremely demanding or have big expectations. But they can make their concerns heard. Address what's bothering you.

Friends in Trouble

So what do you do when good friends are experiencing rough patches? They've gotten fired, been dumped, or are dealing with a health scare or even a death. They're super needy or are perhaps even abusing themselves. Surely these aren't the most positive and healthy types of people to be around.

But here's the thing: Because you've built a strong emotional foundation by cutting out the bad people from your life and surrounding yourself with only the good, you can certainly handle putting yourself out there to help friends in these situations.

That's called being a good friend.

Over the years, I've gotten friends and family to the best health-care professionals when they were sick and others to the best lawyers when in trouble. I've rescued family and friends from debt on many occasions and have had enough people living in spare bedrooms that you'd think I ran a bed-and-breakfast. In turn, I have had friends be as wonderful to me. It all comes back to you.

No matter what, we always have room in the budget—the symbolic budget, consisting of time and energy—to help those we love and those who are good to us. And one of the reasons we always do have room to help the good people in our lives is because those who are toxic do not take our precious time away.

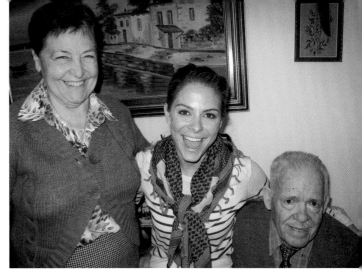

I love visiting my aunt Eleni and uncle Niko in Greece.

EveryGirl Family

I am blessed to have amazing parents and some wonderful aunts, uncles, and cousins, too, all of whom would be there for me at the drop of a hat. I also have my family in Los Angeles, made up of my partner, my dearest friends, and my puppies. In this difficult, sometimes cruel business I'm in, they are my strength and inspiration. Your families should be a positive force in your lives, too.

The same rules we went over with regard to friends apply to your family. This is the hardest thing for most to grasp. We are taught, incorrectly, that family members are more entitled, are allowed to take liberties, and, in the worst cases, get free passes to treat us poorly simply because they are family. No one in this world has that right, not even family.

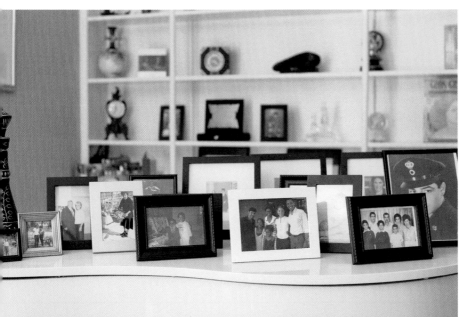

I have framed photos of family and friends around my house to keep them near even though I live so far away.

Having unhealthy relationships and engaging in unhealthy behavior with family members will encourage you to be unhealthy in all of your other relationships—friends, partners, coworkers, and bosses. I have had difficulties with nonfamily relationships because of some of the hardships I endured at the hands of family.

Demand of family members what you would of friends. It will be healthier for you and the family unit overall. My family certainly has its share of demons and bad apples. Luckily, I've worked hard to distance myself from the bad seeds. It took time, some therapy, and a lot of courage, but I'm so much happier and so much more successful since I did.

Standing Up to Family

When family members have wisdom to share and your best interests, at heart, it's wise to consider their advice. But sometimes you have to do what's best for you. My father was dead-set against me moving to LA. After years of obeying him, it was time to exercise my adult right to veto. He stopped talking to me for about a year, which hurt, but in my heart I knew what was best for me and, ironically, what was best for him. Today, nobody has more fun with my success than my dad does. He is so proud, and sorry, too. But it really is okay. The hardship of our temporary fallout only made me tougher and helped prepare me to survive Hollywood—one of the world's toughest businesses.

It doesn't always work out that way. I have a friend who reconnected with her college sweetheart—someone she considered the love of her life. Her family disapproved of him because he was of a different race. The relationship ended. Today, she is in her forties and still single. Sadly, I have too many of these types of stories to share.

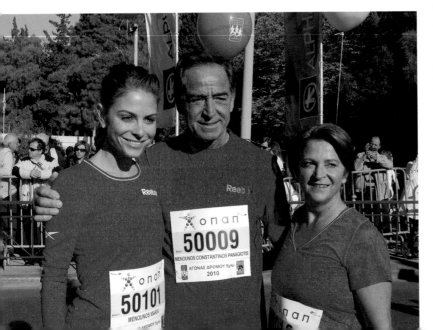

Family or not, at the end of the day, it's your life to live. Consider the advice of loved ones, but live your life how you feel best. If they don't accept your choices, stand your ground. Have courage and conviction—and give it time. If they really love you, they'll come around. Get some therapy, too. It never hurts.

Give Them Some Distance

For those family members who are condescending, undermining, competitive, shameful, or cruel or derail you in any way, the best thing to do is explain to them how they are hurting you. If that doesn't cure the situation, create a polite and healthy distance. This rule especially applies to siblings. They are younger, stronger, and more capable than your parents of changing how they behave.

Repairing Relationships with Long-Lost Family Members

Do family members represent any serious kind of threat to the safety and well-being of your life and family? If so, then you can forgive them in your heart, but remember forgiveness does not always mean reconciliation. If they are no longer a threat, then you can feel free to attempt some form of reconciliation. I caution you that few people in life have the capacity to change. Take reconciliation slowly and be careful. Installing new concrete boundaries and distance with the relationship this time around is always a good idea. If they remain a threat, stand your ground and keep them out. Parents or other family members will pull out all the stops. They may even stop talking to you, the victim, to manipulate you

EveryGirl Extra-Credit Tip: My friend John Comerford has a great positive take on dysfunctional families. He believes God puts us in them to better prepare us for the world!

into relenting. Here's the thing everyone needs to remember: Moms and dads divorce all the time and children have to live with it. If you have to divorce someone from your family for your own well-being, others will learn to live with it, too.

Family Is What You Make It

Having a healthy family *is* crucial. But if God didn't give you a family, then go out and create one for yourself. I don't mean go and start having kids. That's for when you want to be a mother—and when you have a healthy mind-set and lifestyle. I mean that there are certain friends you'll meet who will be your brothers and sisters and maybe even parents and grandparents. The great thing here is that you'll be able to choose them.

Kevin Yorn and Joe Gear are some of the greatest brothers in the

HOW TO HANDLE FAMILY FIGHTS

I asked psychologist Gia Marson about how to fight right with the fam. And here's what she told me:

There are ways to fight that provide more hope for relationship repair. During fights it is best to stick with the current situation rather than bring up past problems. Also, use "I" statements based in how the events make you feel because lots of accusatory "you" statements tend to cause defensiveness. It is equally important to avoid saying things you don't mean, and take a time-out if you think it would provide perspective to either of you.

Once the fight is in the past—by hours, day, or weeks—assess what the relationship means to you. If you hold it as precious, plan to communicate with your friend or family member honestly and calmly while keeping in mind your goal of repairing the relationship. The goal of winning can undermine repair.

During the post-fight dialogue, actually listen. Listening is a skill you can build. When the other person is talking, do not begin preparing your response. Wait, take in what he or she has said, even reflect back your understanding of what you heard, and then respond. Good listening skills will serve you well if you intend to hold onto relationships over time. And finally, saying you're sorry or offering forgiveness is often an element of relationship repair. When you say you're sorry or offer your forgiveness, though, be sure you mean it.

world. Alyssa Wallerce, Meredith Ahern, and Rachel Zalis are three of the best sisters. And these are just a few of my siblings! Some I grew up with, and some I met when I moved to LA. Like my diverse set of friends, they are Jewish, Catholic, Protestant, gay, black, Greek, blue-collar, white-collar, and every other background in between. But they are people who root for me and relate to my life. They are people I call upon when I'm in trouble, and I'm blessed to have them. Remarkably, and to my point, they are not part of my biological family, but they are family in every true sense of the word.

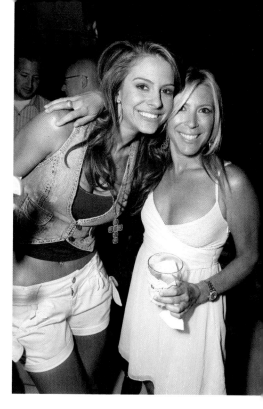

My best friend Rachel Zalis and me at one of my birthday parties.

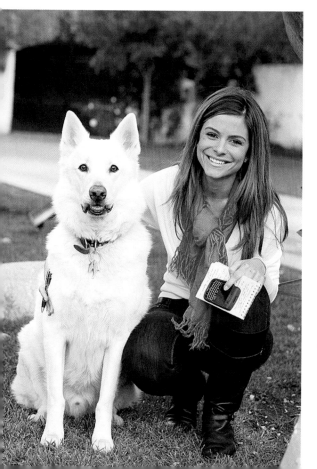

We may have ups and downs with friends and family, but Apollo will always be waiting at home for me with a smile! Dogs are gifts from God.

CHAPTER TEN

EveryGirl in Love

Dating

I've made my share of mistakes, as have so many of my girlfriends. We often just get the whole dating thing wrong. Allow me to share some thoughts and experiences.

Keven and me chilling at home in our screening room.

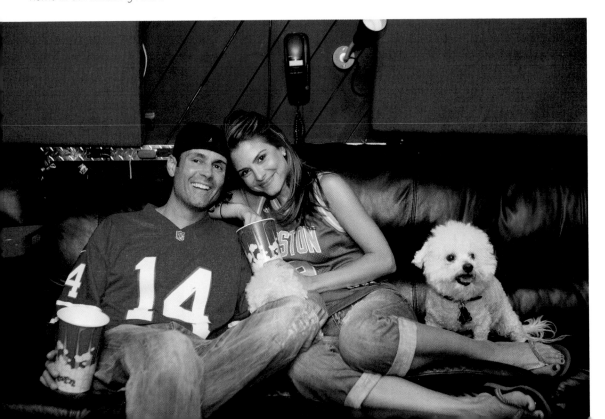

Maria Answers Your Most Pressing Dating Questions

Can you ask him out?

Absolutely! But be casual about it. Don't make it all official. Say, *Hey, Matt, do you want to grab a bite to eat or get coffee sometime?* If you make it casual, it's more likely he'll accept. He won't be thinking about an official date and all the baggage that goes along with it. When you do get him out, just see how it goes from there.

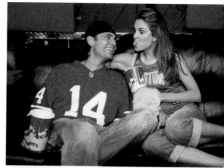

Should I date for money?

My man was bankrupt and living in a basement when we began dating. In the ideal relationship, you'll be a team who will work together to earn lots of money. We did. You don't want a deadbeat or screwup though. Along with treating me well, my guy was responsible, with a strong work ethic. Expect the same from your guy.

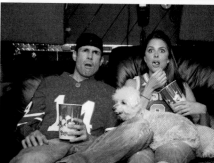

How do I know if he's a bum?

Beware of guys who can't hold a job or have no career aspirations. This type of behavior reveals mountains about who they are as human beings. It shows a lack of discipline, commitment, care, and focus. These drawbacks will hurt you in the long run.

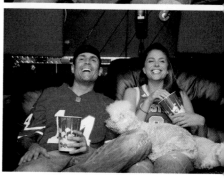

How do I keep my girlfriends out of my love life?

I love my girlfriends, but I've learned *not* to talk to them about my relationship. They're not in the relationship. They're not dating and living with my guy, so they can't possibly fully understand what's right or wrong. It just makes a mess later. The only time to bring a girlfriend in is for a breakup or if you've been seriously hurt. But don't be in denial, either. If your family and friends all have bad things to say about your guy—take an honest look at your relationship.

How can I stop obsessing over him?

In our technology age, it's common to call, e-mail, and text your boyfriend . . . ten trillion times a day. *Stop.* Stop obsessing about every unreturned text, and don't follow it up with three more of them. A simple rule is to take turns. You send a text, e-mail, or leave a phone message and then *wait* until he tosses one back.

Should you . . . on the first date?

No. Never. Guys do like the chase and, deep down, generally want relationships (real ones) with women who are more traditional. If you spend that first night in bed, it might end up being your last with him.

EveryGirl Extra-Credit Tip: Guys love it when you don't talk during sporting events. It's not that you have to shut up entirely, but imagine him talking all the way through the next *Sex and the City* film.

Maria's Guy Rules

Give and Take

You dragged him to that chick flick or nephew's birthday party and now he wants to watch football or baseball. Don't whine and say you hate sports or watch and nag and ask, "When is this *ever* going to be over?" Guys hate that. It's annoying. Instead, get into it with him. I once hated watching basketball, baseball, and football, but for my guy I bit the bullet. Now, I'm obsessed with sports! Some of our most fun times are watching games together, and we look forward to different upcoming seasons.

Don't Expect Big Gifts

The key here is to not expect big gifts when you're dating, even for a big event like an anniversary or a birthday. Don't put that pressure on your guy or your relationship. We're living through crazy economic times

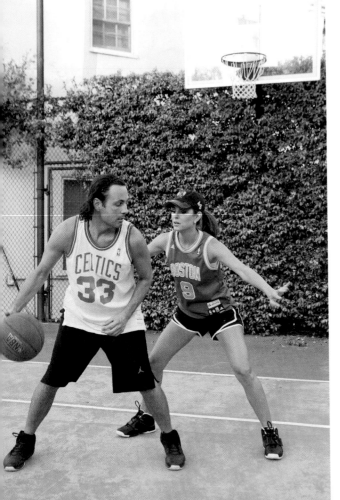

We love to play basketball. You obviously know our favorite team.

and there are more important things to expect in a relationship: loyalty, dedication, respect, and consideration. So long as he or she remembers the day and takes the effort to make it special, that's all you need.

What to Do About His Female Friends

Don't freak if he has a good female friend who is just a friend. If he wanted to be with her romantically, he would be. But as your relationship grows, he should be confiding in you and spending more time with you than her. If he's not, it's a problem, but don't come off as insecure or as a psycho. Just say, "I'm a bit uncomfortable."

Don't Ask Him (Early on), "Where Is This Going?"

Do not decide in your mind that you will bail if you don't have a ring in six months. This puts too much pressure on him . . . and you. Plus, these timetables people create don't work anymore. Spend as much time as possible getting to know each other and see how you connect and bond. Quick marriages can mean quicker divorces.

Oh, and Let Him Hang with His Boys

Don't be the girl who bans guy night, because he will just feel like he's in a prison cell. If you ban this, then he will want to go even more . . . and maybe even tell you a white lie, like he has to work late. You can't control someone else, and you want him to love you and not resent you. And P.S., don't be afraid to become one of the boys, either. Become interested in his hobbies and he'll eventually want to spend more time with you than the boys!

Don't Live in the Bathroom

Obviously this doesn't apply to occasions like weddings and big affairs, but for the day-to-day stuff, guys hate it. Find ways and some looks to help speed up getting ready. Putting your hair in a ponytail and

EveryGirl Extra-Credit Tip: There are classes and seminars out there specifically designed to teach women about sports so they can enjoy watching them with the guys. Go online and find one to take with girlfriends in your area.

Keven and I are laughing at Artie Lange's performance in Serial Buddies.

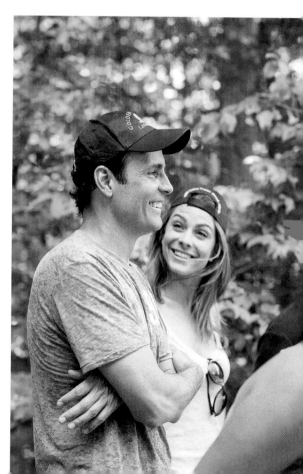

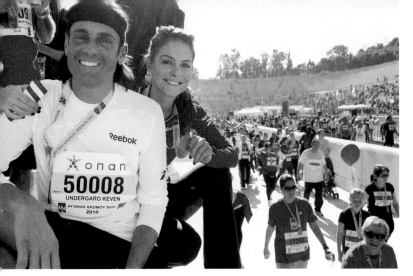

Keven and I ran in the 5k at the 2,500th anniversary of the Greek marathon.

applying some foundation and a little mascara doesn't take long.

Be Creative

Put little *I love you* notes in his socks or in his car. It's a little thing that is a big deal.

Listen to Him

This might sound simple, but really listen to him. Look him in the eye. Hold his hand. And listen. Guys keep more pain and stress inside than we do, and it's not healthy. By encouraging him to express his feelings, he will feel better and the two of you will become closer.

Get on the Forty-Year Plan

In my relationship, I would leave half-empty water bottles all over the house. It was minor, to me. However, minor things add up to major problems over the span of forty-plus years—the time many of us in long-term relationships hope to be together. My partner sat me down and explained that this annoyed him. He told me that *he* was on the forty-year plan— that *he* wanted to be together in forty years, and that this thing I was doing was driving him bonkers and would really put a strain on us in the long run. He also reminded me about the things he had changed about himself for my sake. He used to leave cabinet doors and drawers open all over the house, which annoyed me. When I let him know, he stopped. All this gave me great perspective. He wasn't just nagging me or bitching; instead, he was trying to help us stay together. I made the adjustment. That's another key to staying in love. You need to make adjustments constantly.

Some Shortcomings Are Better to Just Accept

You should never accept things like neglect, cheating, or abuse of any kind, but there are lesser shortcomings that are just better to accept. If you accept some of these shortcomings openly, your partner should, and will, be more likely to do the same. As I said, couples can spend years battling over minutiae until they absolutely hate each other.

You Are "Partners!"

At the end of the day, you're not lovers as much as you're partners, arm in arm, fighting the battles and experiencing the joys in life.

Roles

And because you are equal partners, don't be insecure about assuming roles that are necessary to make the partnership work. My old neighbor Margie knew it was *her* role to run *all* household matters and to keep her partner healthy. His role was to bring home the bacon. This goes for man *or* woman. If you're both breadwinners, then you should divide work and duties in a way that's equal and fair to both. The work duties and roles you assume are about whatever's best for the team and partnership. Remember, each role is 50 percent of the partnership, making you equals and neither better than the other.

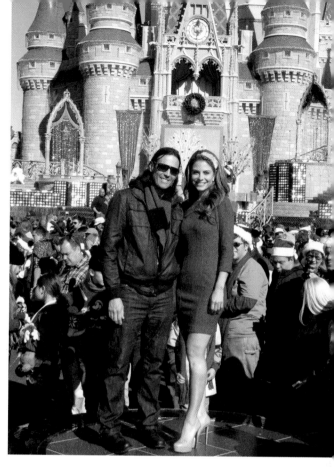

I hosted the 2009 ABC Christmas Day Parade in Disney World. Here I am with Keven in front of Cinderella's castle.

The Couple That Works Together Stays Together

When my dad cleaned nightclubs, my mom was right there working with him. She learned a great deal about repairs as a result and she was also there to help monitor my dad's blood sugar. Dad got done faster, and they made more money as a result. There are all sorts of ways to work together. Sometimes, it's just listening to your partner's work woes and giving advice.

Keep Things Fresh

Remember when you were first dating? You were sure to have fresh breath, look your best, be spontaneous and polite. Yet over time we begin

EveryGirl Extra-Credit Tip: Move the TV. Studies show that having a TV in the bedroom dramatically decreases your sex life, which increases your chances of splitting up.

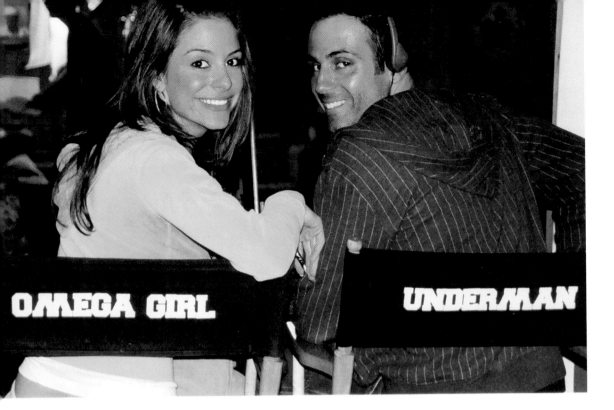

OMEGA GIRL

UNDERMAN

Keven and me on set producing/directing a short film called Longtime Listener.

EveryGirl Extra-Credit Tip: Try establishing routines, such as *We're going to kiss each other good night every night* or *We're going to have a specified and recurring date night every Saturday.*

to care less about our appearance, abandon spontaneity, and ditch the etiquette that we used to show one another. We stop trying. Both parties are usually too tired from their respective long days, but that's when relationships get old. This *for sure* relates to your sex life, too. Invest the time and the effort in keeping things fresh, and the relationship will be far better off in the long run.

Relationships Need to Stay in *Kaizen,* Too

No matter how good things are for you as a couple, keep challenging yourselves as to how the relationship could be better.

Build It into Your New Year Plan

When you do your New Year plan, you and your partner can go over couple plans for the upcoming year. A few examples:

- We're going to take a vacation this year.
- We're going to take ballroom dancing lessons.
- I'm going to put the dishes away, and you're going to replace empty toilet paper rolls.

New Family First, Old Family Second

I've seen marriages crumble due to the fact that people can't separate from their nuclear families. Partners who put Mom, Dad, and their siblings first over life partners are setting the marriage up for failure. Your life partner comes first.

Marry Your Best Friend

If you don't listen to any of the advice I've written, then at least listen to this one. Before you marry someone, ask yourself if he is truly your best friend. In addition to being attracted to him, is he your best friend in the entire world? Looks fade, as does physical attraction. It's not a cliché; it's true: What will always remain is your friendship.

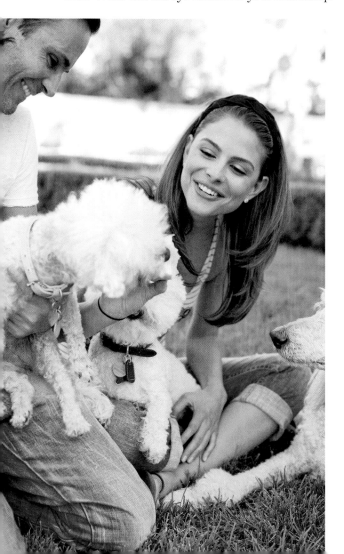

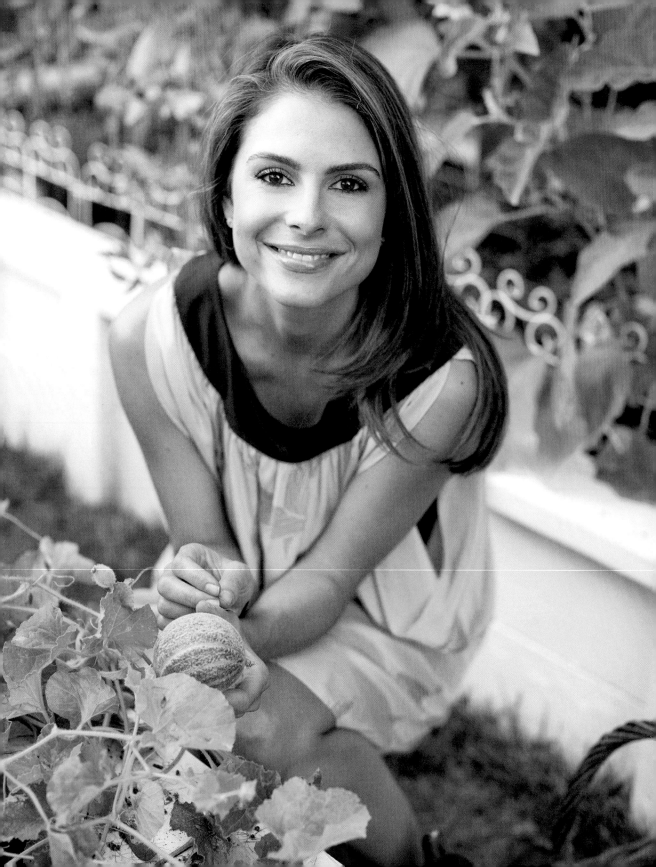

part four

HEALTH AND THE EVERYGIRL

EVERYONE SAYS HEALTH IS THE MOST IMPORTANT THING IN LIFE BECAUSE IT IS. No matter how rich or good-looking someone is, if their health goes everything is meaningless. I think through modern medicine many of us will live longer. However, it's the quality of life that we'll have in those later years that I question. What good is living if you are in pain, feeble, or immobile? I don't know about you, but in my later years, I want to be able to enjoy the fruits of my earnings and my life in general. Being mindful of your health now will best ensure quality of life later. I wasn't always mindful, as you'll soon learn, but I got better. I grow more mindful of my health every day and I hope you do, too.

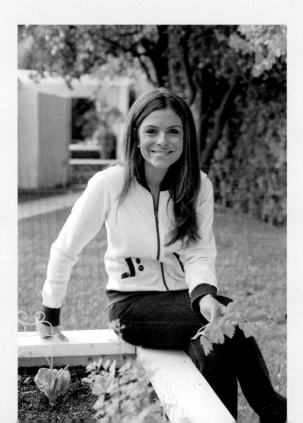

EveryGirl Loses Weight

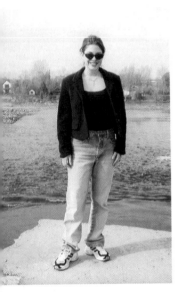

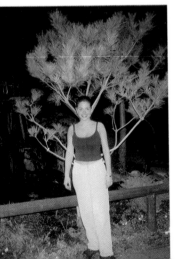

Growing up, I was thin. The diet in my home was different than most people's because my dad was a type-1 diabetic and because of the way my parents grew up. They came from small villages in the mountains of Greece, where they ate meat once a year and lived mainly on the fruits and vegetables they farmed from their gardens. And that's mostly what we ate—a diet rich in fresh fruits and vegetables, some from our summer garden, and low in carbohydrates and sugar, due to my dad's diabetes.

I didn't know what a bagel was until late in high school. Waffles? No clue. There were no chips, no ice cream, and no sugary cereals. I was raised thinking Grape-Nuts and Bran Flakes were yummy. Dinner items were lentils, stuffed vegetables, and beans from the garden. Dessert was fruit. The only soda we ever had was diet, and that's only because Dad used to drink it.

While my dad was concerned that I would get diabetes, too, at other times I remember my parents telling me I was too skinny. My dad would come home from work sometimes with the biggest chocolate bars he could find and give them to me so I could put on weight.

I started out freshman year in high school as a size 3. Working at Dunkin' Donuts (how I loved Dunkin' Donuts, and still do!) probably contributed, but every year from then on, I grew a size, and by senior year I was a size 8. I was definitely comfortable with my appearance. Even though I was told I was too short for a modeling career, I par-

In these photos I was a size 12–14. It wasn't that I thought I looked bad, I just didn't have the energy I needed to work in the news. My diet was also very unhealthy.

ticipated in small fashion shows and even did some print work.

If I weren't comfortable at a size 8, I surely wouldn't have competed in the Miss Massachusetts Teen USA pageant, where I had to don a swimsuit. And for any of you girls who think you need to be a size 2 to be attractive, maybe you'll change your mind after I tell you that I actually won that pageant.

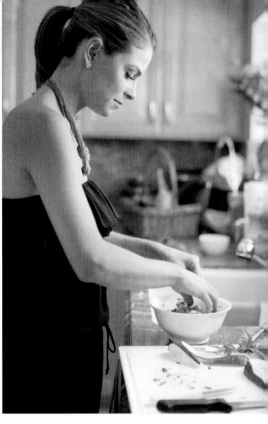

"Sexy bodies come in all shapes and sizes. Being healthy is important, so you don't want to be too overweight. But don't freak out if you're not a size 2. Nobody is really a size 2, except maybe ten-year-olds!"

—Glynis Costin,
InStyle *magazine West Coast bureau chief*

My weight gain started in high school, but it was during freshman year in college when it began to get unhealthy. I didn't gain the freshman fifteen. Instead, I gained the freshman forty! Between my roommate Tara's M&M'S jar and our late-night pizza orders—not to mention the school cafeteria—it was inevitable.

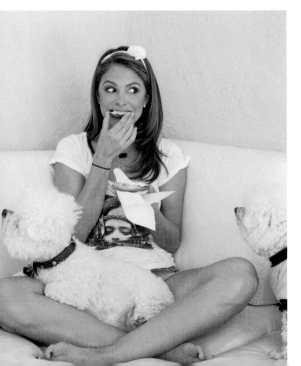

At the cafeteria, there were endless rows of all-you-can-eat fries, steak-and-cheese subs, sandwich melts, cakes, pies, pudding, and ice cream. These were all foods I'd never been allowed to eat or ever been offered—and certainly not in such an abundance. It was all there for the taking, with no one to stop me, and it was too much for me to handle. I ate it . . . all!

Coming from a home where junk food was nonexistent, it was complete culture shock for my body and for me. Soon enough I was almost a size 14 . . . and growing. Again, I don't remember really thinking I looked that bad, and I still don't think I did.

Members of my family felt otherwise. Every time I came home from college, aunts, uncles, and cousins had something mean to say. Having watched me during my early teenage years participating in the fashion shows and in the pageants, they would smile, wave their hands, to imitate a beauty queen, and say, "Remember this?" and then laugh. It all really hurt—enough for me to buy a gallon of ice cream and hide in the garage, where I would consume it all, defiantly.

EveryGirl Extra-Credit Tip: When your family is on you about your weight, politely say, "I appreciate your concern, but you're only hurting me and making things worse." If they continue to badger you, repeat the phrase. If they still continue, walk away. If they bring it up again in the future, act as if you didn't hear them. If you're super close, sit them down and explain to them in more detail how you feel.

A Maria Moment: Thank You, J.Lo, and Beyoncé

Despite the shaming from my family, when I returned to school, I maintained a healthy degree of self-confidence. J.Lo and Beyoncé definitely helped matters, as booties were being revered. In the era of celebrities who are vapid and reckless, J.Lo and Beyoncé do not get enough credit. And let me vouch for them personally. Sometimes when I interview beautiful women, they can be competitive and downright catty, but J.Lo and Beyoncé are two beautiful women who are always sweet. Like me, both are self-made and from humble roots. They're just good girls who come from good families, and they do a lot for women.

At school, I continued to thrive, having won Emerson College's EVVY Award for broadcast journalism. Emerson was attended by the likes of Jay Leno, Denis Leary, Henry Winkler, Norman Lear, and countless other names in show business, and I was the very first freshman in the school's seventy-five-year history to win the award. For any of you who think you need to be a size 0 to be on camera or to be beautiful, I won this award when I was a size 14.

Needless to say I was feeling proud—all one-hundred-fifty-plus pounds or so of me. But I began to notice that I didn't have the energy that

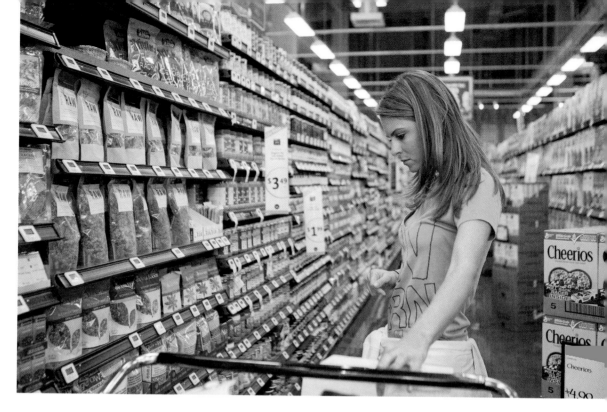

I did when I was thinner. All I'd ever heard from teachers about working in TV was that it requires a high level of energy and stamina. You have to be prepared to work eighteen-hour days. My decreased energy was beginning to impede my lifelong dream. Also, the ravaging effects of diabetes were all too familiar. When I learned that my overeating and weight gain were putting me at greater risk to contract the disease, the writing was on the wall: I had to take my health more seriously.

I tried things like Slim-Fast shakes, the grapefruit diet, and the Coffee Diet, but each lasted barely a day. I loved to eat and just couldn't stop. Pills were out of the question, too. I knew they weren't the answer, as they would negatively affect my health in another way, and thankfully, I hate swallowing pills! I opted to take a long-term approach to it—just cutting back a little on portions. It was easier for my will power to handle. Little did I know that it was not only the healthiest way to lose the weight but also the best way to ensure I wouldn't gain it back—and I haven't so far!

I always try to choose healthy snacks at the supermarket, so when I'm hungry, I grab nuts instead of potato chips.

EveryGirl Extra-Credit Tip: Don't allow your weight to pull the plug on your dreams. Get in shape for your health, but remember you can pretty much do anything—at any weight.

How to Lose Weight

EveryGirl Extra-Credit Tip: The longer you take to gradually lose the weight, the longer it will take to put it back on and the more realistic your chances of remaining in shape. Give yourself, enough to lose the total weight you want to lose.

Step 1: Set a Goal

It always helps to have your weight loss goal tied to a specific event. Some people need to get in shape in order to run the city marathon, and others need to lose weight for their upcoming class reunions. In my case, it was the Miss Massachusetts USA pageant. It was January 1999, and I decided I would set a goal for myself to compete that November.

Sponsorship money was due in the earlier half of the year, and I definitely wasn't going to waste the entrance fee if I wasn't seriously going to lose the weight. So I said to myself, If you don't start losing in the first few months of 1999, you won't be competing in November.

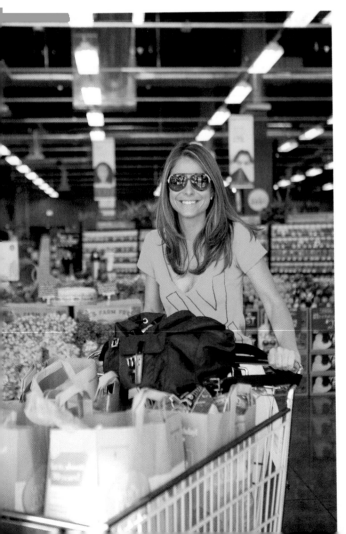

Step 2: Write Down Everything That Goes into Your Mouth (You Might Be Surprised!)

After you've set a target goal for your weight loss, the second step involves writing in your weight loss journal. I journaled everything I ate each day for a week, including little things like gum and breath mints. When you do this, you'll be amazed to see all the food you *really* consume. I saw how much I was eating and was literally stunned. I think we all lie to ourselves about what we really eat in a day. It helped get me on track. I've included samples of my food journals in the appendix.

At the end of the week, reevaluate your diet. Where are your problem areas? I learned my biggest problem was carbs. I was eating tons of them. Cutting carbs therefore became my focus.

I like to stock up on a full cart of fresh, tasty, and healthy things to eat.

My Diet at Its Worst

By the time I decided to do the Miss Mass USA pageant and to lose weight, my diet had reached its worst. I would eat a large bagel and cream cheese for breakfast; a large steak-and-cheese sandwich with lots of french fries for lunch; pizza for dinner; and ice cream, candy, and assorted junk in between. I was so obsessed with Brown Sugar Cinnamon Pop-Tarts that, to this day, I won't eat them for fear the taste will get me readdicted! At dinner, I indulged in the more fattening foods, such as pizza—I would down an entire one by myself. Two hours after dinner, three Eggo waffles were my dessert.

Eating became a game to me. I started to compete with guys to see who could eat the most, and regrettably, I always won. At my heaviest, I was one hundred and fifty-five pounds.

EveryGirl Extra-Credit Tip: Keep a food journal as you are cutting back to help chart your progress. You may want to write down what exercises you did along with what you ate each day. This can include the little things that aren't so little, like parking far away and walking across a big parking lot. When you see four days go by with nothing in the exercise department, it's time to move it! Conversely, when you see the four days that you did work out, you'll be proud.

Step 3: Cut Back . . . Slowly

Now that you know just what you're eating, it's time to cut back, *slowly*, starting with those trouble areas. Instead of seven slices of pizza for one meal, I would eat six. Even with this tiny adjustment, it was still difficult to say no. But over time, it became less painful, and then I knew I could cut down to five slices.

When I finally cut down to three slices, I started to incorporate a salad. It was a healthier way to feel full and made it easier to keep cutting back. If you cut out your favorite foods cold turkey, it's more painful and harder to do. Don't think of it as *I can never have a chocolate chip cookie for the rest of my life*. It's about eating less.

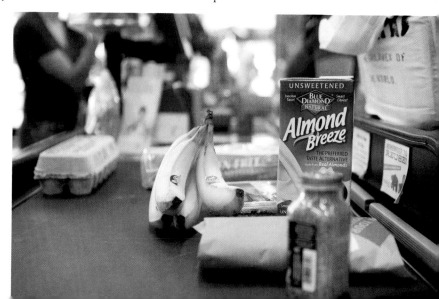

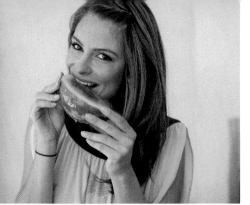

EveryGirl Extra-Credit Tip: While trying to lose weight, the one word I never uttered was "diet." Don't even tell others you're trying to lose weight. It's more pressure. More pressure only increases your chances of failure. This is just about making some better choices in your eating habits.

Step 4: To Scale or Not to Scale

Don't weigh yourself for at least three months. Five months into my cutting back, my mom told me she thought I had lost weight. Finally I got on the scale. To my surprise, I had lost twenty pounds, which was enough inspiration for me to keep going! And I didn't get on the scale for another five months.

You'll only risk disappointment, get obsessed with the numbers, put more pressure on yourself, and increase your chance of failure if you check the scale often.

Step 5: Keep Cutting Down

Eventually, I cut my carbs down to one carb serving or item a day, and I chose whether I was going to eat it at breakfast, lunch, or dinner. If pasta was on the menu for dinner . . . well, that was the one carb for the day. I would measure the pasta and have only one cup of it. If I wanted a wrap for lunch, that was my carb. This was a good way to limit my carbs but not cut them out entirely..

DEALING WITH YOUR FAMILY AND THE WEIGHT ISSUE
BY EVERYGIRL EXPERT DR. GAIL SALTZ, PSYCHIATRIST AND PSYCHOANALYST

There are many young women who tell me their parents mean well, but they're "on their case" for various issues, including weight gain. How can you politely ask family members to get off your back?

Let's talk about the weight issue. It's hard for your parents to see you gain weight. To some degree, it's a reflection on them. People want their children to be attractive. It's a case of "I gave birth to you. I want you to look and feel great." There is some degree of truth to the idea that when your weight is under reasonable control you are healthier and perhaps happier. In today's culture, it doesn't help if you're overweight. The problem is how parents talk about weight, because they could make you feel worse. Some young women might even rebel and gain more weight without knowing it. Say to your well-meaning parents, "I know what I weigh. I'm going to do something about it when I'm ready to do something about it. I really need you to keep your thoughts to yourself." Then add, "I know you love me and want the best for me, but what you're saying to me is hurting our relationship."

Step 6: Eat Your Calories— Don't Drink Them

I would chop lemons and push them into jugs of spring water for flavor and drink this in lieu of something else filled with calories. It also makes it tasty, so I *want* to reach for it.

Step 7: Get a Good Burn from Foods!

I made myself all kinds of different egg-white omelets each morning, too, but the very first thing I would eat was a grapefruit, which I had heard burns fat.

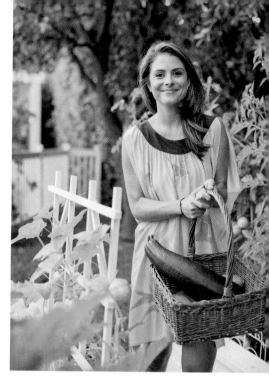

I get a lot of my fresh veggies from my garden.

EATING ACTION ITEMS

- Drink eight to ten glasses of pure spring water a day.
- Omit any sugary sodas.
- Don't keep junk food in your house! If it's not there, you won't eat it.
- If you must snack between meals (and try not to), munch on carrots. They'll fill you up.
- Eat small meals more often—say four to five smaller meals a day, in lieu of three bigger ones. This is better for your metabolism and may curb snack cravings.
- Keep a little bit of fat in your diet because your body needs it. Use extra-virgin olive oil for cooking and make your own salad dressings with it and a wide variety of specialty vinegars. A little bit of coconut milk is also a great healthy fat.
- End your eating day after dinner. Take a nice bath, read a book, surf the net, and stay out of the kitchen. Try not to eat after 6 P.M.
- Eat only when you're hungry. We are conditioned to think we need breakfast in the morning, lunch at noon, and so on. If you're not hungry—don't eat.
- If you're hungry, have some hot water or chamomile tea. It's filling and will curb your appetite.

STOP DRINKING THESE BEVERAGES IF YOU WANT TO LOSE WEIGHT

- Sugary cola, which is packed with high-fructose corn syrup—another word for sugar.
- Fancy coffee drinks loaded with sugar and whipped cream. They can top out at eight hundred calories.
- Alcoholic drinks with fruit-juice mixers and added sugars. These include flavored martinis, piña coladas, margaritas, wine, and wine coolers. Vodka (in moderation) is the one form of alcohol that's lower in carbs.

Step 8: Don't Forget Dessert

I was never on a diet so I never deprived myself. If I wanted a cookie or two, I had them. I would just look at the back for the fat and calorie content, and only ate what it said the serving was. I ate slowly and savored each bite and didn't reach for more. I had my taste. I also kept carb-smart ice cream on hand for those nights I wanted a cool, refreshing treat. Try Greek yogurt with some berries for a low-cal option.

Growing my own food has given me a deeper appreciation for what I put into my body.

Step 9: Rejoice! Success!

By November, I had lost forty pounds. I felt like I was a little too thin at that point and, soon after, gained a few pounds back to get to a good place. My energy was back and I was breathing better. Reflecting on that time, I think of how great it was that I lost all of that weight on my own. I identified my problem area, cut back, set myself up for success by not telling anyone, didn't try to cheat or take shortcuts that would only be temporary solutions, and was patient. Follow these rules for your own weight-loss success. Believe me, if I can do it, so can you!

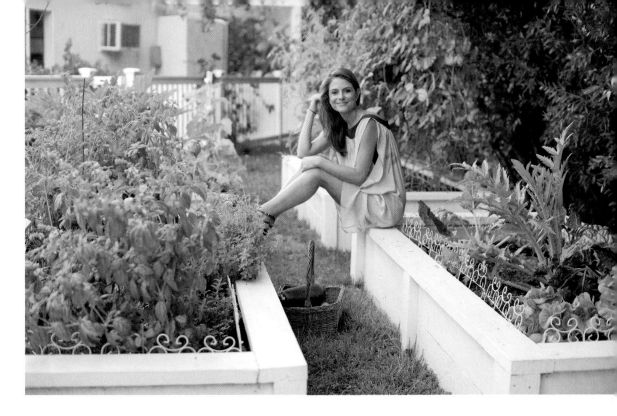

Stop Trying to Look Like Her—Whoever She Is

There's always someone who will be more toned or thinner, so it's pointless to compare; you'll just end up feeling defeated. We are all different, and that's a good thing.

If you are obsessing over your weight, I implore you to change the way you think. Be proud of your curves and of what you look like. If you do, you'll radiate a confidence that everyone will feel.

FOODS THAT GIVE YOU A GOOD BURN

- Grapefruit on an empty stomach
- Hot sauces of any kind
- Jalapeños
- Vinegar
- Tabasco sauce
- Basically anything spicy!
  Note: Enjoy these in moderation!

It's all about the attitude.

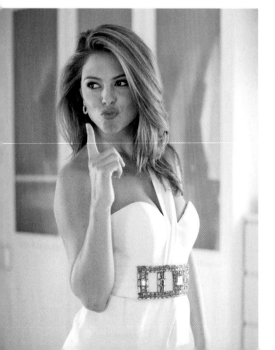

Get a High from Saying No!

I learned how to get a high from saying no to food. If I was at a friend's or family member's home and they offered me dessert or extras, I would politely say no. You'll notice that people are always impressed when you have the willpower. This empowered me. It gave me a sense of accomplishment and was a helpful tool in my losing weight.

My Bottom Line Is Health

After my long diet journey—through the heavy carbs I consumed during college, the fast food I consumed at the beginning of my career (more on that later), and my full-circle embrace of the fresh-fare diet I was initially raised on—I'm now at a comfortable place. At five-eight, I weigh in somewhere between 125 and 130 pounds. I wear a size 4 in dresses for the most part because I have a small waist. With jeans, I'm usually a 28, but sometimes I go up to a 29 if I put on a few pounds, which I still do from time to time. The one thing I don't do is freak out about it.

The main thing I'd like to stress is that it's all about health. When it's all said and done, it's not about being skinny, it's about being healthy. Also, know that no one is perfect. We all have areas we can be insecure about. I have friends who most women would hate to hear complain about their bodies, and they obsess about their weight constantly. Every day it's "Am I fat?" or "Can you see I gained weight?" (and by the way, the answer is usually no). Kim Kardashian is just as confident when she's gained a few pounds as when she has lost them. She owns her curves. That ownership and that confidence is what makes her so sexy. In addition, a lot of men don't really like skinny women. I recently was at a big movie star's home and he and his male friends were going on and on about how the girls in Hollywood are too skinny, how they gross them out, and how they wished there were more curvy girls like Kim or Beyoncé. I asked, "So all these girls in the fashion pages don't do it for you?" They all replied, "Too skinny." The curvier the better, they said. I remember them positively drooling over Ice T's wife, Coco. Last, there's always someone who will be more toned or thinner or whatever, so it's pointless to compare. Just own your body and be confident—everyone will notice you and not your weight. Confidence gives you the strongest sex appeal of all and, in the end, your health is the most vital.

One way to encourage yourself to love your body is to use self-talk focused on health instead of self-talk based on criticism. After all, health is a value most of us hold. In general, girls who view exercise as a behavior that improves health, rather than as a punishment for having a body shape or size that does not match up to a thin ideal, stay more mo-tivated to make sustained, positive health choices. Remind yourself that your body is a means to living a meaningful life, not the goal of life.

–Dr. Gia Marson, psychologist

Kim Kardashian is a great friend. Like me, she owns her curves and I thank her for being a great example to all of us.

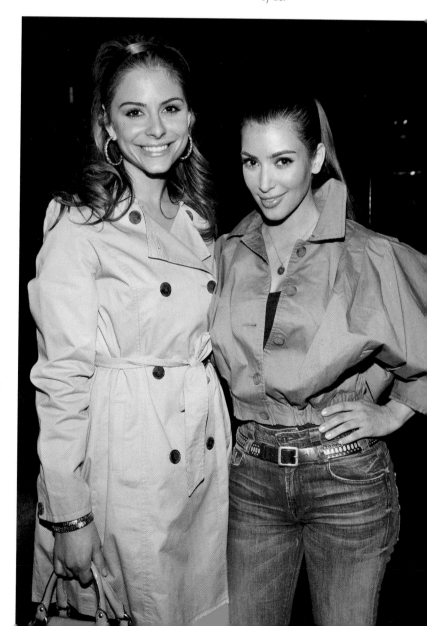

EveryGirl Stays Fit

When I was thirteen, a card came in the mail for the Miss Massachusetts Teen USA beauty pageant. I thought participating in the pageant was a step in the right direction toward having a career in the entertainment industry, but my parents vetoed the idea. Being on a stage in heels and a bathing suit isn't really big on a Greek immigrant father's list of "can-dos" for his daughter. Still, I kept the pageant invitation card and at fourteen was ready to ask permission again. This time, attacking an old problem in a new way, I reached out for help to someone older and wiser, my cousin Anthony.

Anthony acted like a manager to me in those days. He believed in me and was always willing to help me fulfill my dreams. My parents trusted Anthony, so when he told them I should enter the pageant, they agreed. And I won! The experience and my success suddenly had others taking notice.

One of those people was a man by the name of Harry Bouras, who ran the Channel—that nightclub in Boston that I'd been cleaning with my parents. Harry scored me a meeting with this amazing photographer named Jean Renard, a man who was also Niki Taylor's manager at the time. Jean told me that, at five-eight, I was a little on the shorter end to model. However, if I wanted to make a go of it, I should begin working out with a trainer to tone up. Always one to heed good advice, I began working out with a personal trainer named Ina Krueger. Anthony paid for the sessions, and I worked

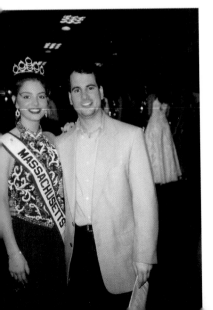

Me with my cousin Anthony, who got me into working out.

out with her two to three times a week. I had to travel to Boston for the workouts, and Ina trained me like she would a bodybuilder. It was hard, heavy lifting, but I learned a lot and built good "muscle memory."

Your Workout Routine

One Training Session Is All It Takes

So with Ina, I built up some muscle memory for sure, but I tapered off from working out altogether. I couldn't afford to continue the sessions, and the gym was just too far a commute. From the age of sixteen on, I experienced my previously discussed weight gains and losses and didn't resume working out seriously till I was twenty-one, when I decided to compete in the pageant. Once again, my cousin Anthony helped. This time, he paid for me to have one session with a local trainer, Debbie Maida. We met, and she put me on a simple workout plan.

EveryGirl Extra-Credit Tip: Need extra encouragement? Ask a friend to be your gym buddy.

There was no need for a celebrity trainer and no need to hire someone to train me three times a week. All it took was one fifty-dollar session with Debbie for me to gather all the knowledge I needed. Debbie wrote out a general circuit program that included jumping rope, push-ups, and sit-ups, as well as triceps extensions, curls, shoulder presses, upright and one-arm rows, leg lifts, step-ups, squats, and lunges—all with light handheld weights. I would get my cardio through exercising on the elliptical machine. Check out the exact workout Deb gave me in the appendix.

Your goal is to find a trainer near where you live and hire him or her for one session. Make sure the trainer knows that you want a circuit routine that you can do on your own. Tell the trainer to tailor it to the equipment you have to work with—a professional gym or whatever you have at home. And have your trainer write the workout down for you. You can use this workout on your own from then on.

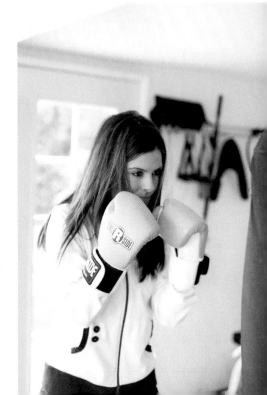

In time, return to the trainer if you feel like the workout is getting stale. Or, to save money, ask the trainer if you can split the session with a friend. My best friend Rachel and I do it all the time, and it's a fun way to see each other.

My Workout Routine

I joined a gym that was, conveniently, five minutes from my house, and I worked out three to five days a week, following Debbie's plan. If it's hard at first, just stick with it. I used to pile magazines up and would occupy my time reading and looking at pictures.

Here's the workout my Los Angeles fitness specialist Andrea Orbeck taught me. I save time and money by doing this at home on my own. Well, Bon Jovi is always there with me . . . does that count? He keeps me livin' on a prayer! Ha-ha.

I do two sets of twenty for each move.

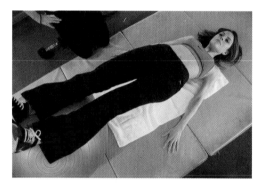 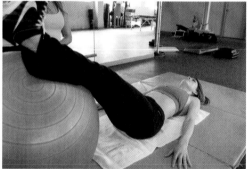

Supine Ball Hip Lifts on Ball: Lying on a mat, place your heels on a ball, shoulder width apart and hands at sides, palms facing down for balance. Grip the ball with your heels, toes facing toward the ceiling, and lift the glutes until the body is in a plank position. Maintain stability without rolling off the ball. For an easier movement, place the ball under the calf muscles instead of the heels.

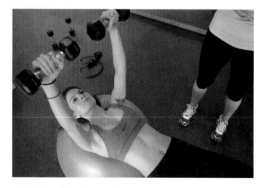 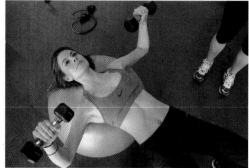

Ball Flies for Pecs: Using the ball as a bench, lower your body into a bridge position until your head is on the ball and your butt is raised and contracted so that you look like a tabletop. With weights in hand, press your hands forward into the air (think of a mummy sleepwalking) with your palms facing toward your knees. Using your pecs, lower your elbows to a 90-degree angle, or until the backs of your arms are touching the ball, then press the hands back up to the starting position.

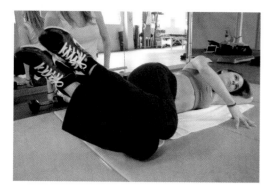 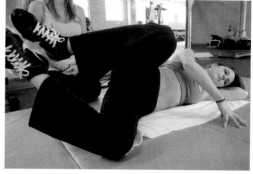

Lateral Clams: Lying on your side with your knees and ankles together, lift both ankles into the air. Open the top knee with the feet still together. Keep the heels together, both feet rotated into the air.

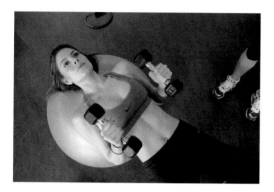 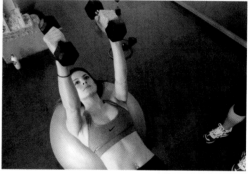

Close Grip Press on Ball (Triceps and Pecs): Lying on the ball in a bridge position, follow the same movements as the Ball Flies for Pecs, the difference being in the grip. Here, palms are facing each other and the arms are lowered to the ribs. Keep the hips up during the movement and the elbows close to the sides.

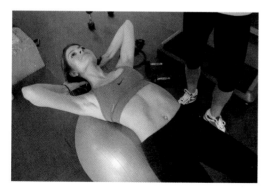 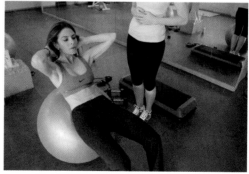

Ball Abs: Sit on the ball on top of a nonslip surface. Walk your feet away from you as you lie on the ball until the lower back is on the center of the ball. With your hands behind your neck, contract your abs and slide your ribs into your hips as you would in a sit-up. Press your lower back into the ball as you lower your shoulders parallel to the floor. If you feel discomfort in your back in this movement, lower your hips closer to the floor.

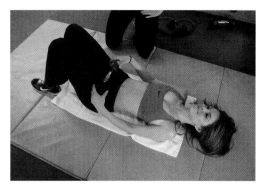 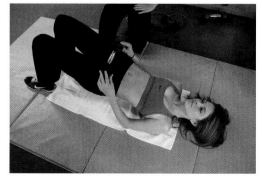

Reverse Butt Bridges: Lying on your back, knees bent with a weight across your hips, push your hips into the air and using the glutes, slowly lower back to the floor. Keep your knees in alignment with your hips and shoulders.

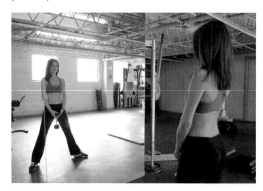 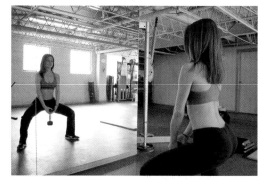

Pile Squat with Dumbbell: Stand in a squat position with your hands extended in front, holding at least a 10-pound dumbbell, and with your knees and toes turned out. Squat by lowering your butt into a second position ballet squat. Feel your leg and butt muscles as you lower yourself and use them to press through the heels and slowly return to a standing position.

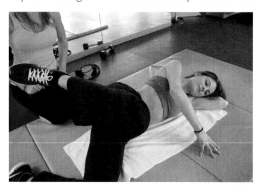 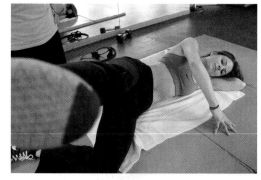

Clam with Knee Extensions: Lie on your side with your hips and knees stacked, shoulders pulled back, and head lying on the bent arm closest to the floor. Contract your gluteus and raise your top knee (think of a clam opening) toward the ceiling without moving your hips, pause and extend the knee like you are kicking. Bend the knee back and return the knee slowly to the start position. This is a modification of the clam as you have to maintain a glute contraction while you straighten and bend your knee in the air.

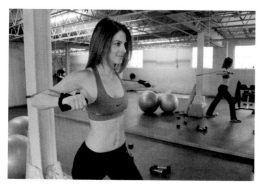 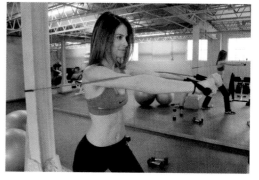

Standing Band Chest Flies: Hook the band to a secure place and with a staggered stance for balance, grip handles at your ribs. Walk far enough away from the anchor to generate tension, grip starting at shoulder height, elbows bent at a 90-degree angle. Press the hands out and in front of the chest. Using a slow and controlled motion, return the hands to the start position.

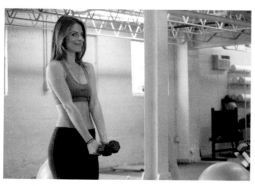 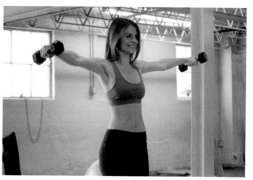

Standing Dumbbell Lateral Raises: Stand with a strong posture, feet hip width apart and hips tucked under, and hold either 3- or 5-pound dumbbells. Slightly bend the elbows and lift chest. Using your shoulders, raise your slightly bent arms parallel to the height of your shoulders. Refrain from shrugging your shoulders toward your ears.

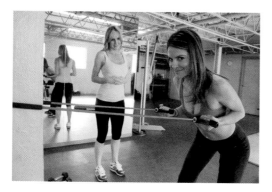 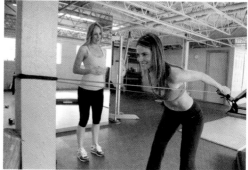

Bent-over Triceps Extensions with Band: Anchor the band to a source and stand with tension in the band, elbows bent at sides. Hinge over at the hips, knees slightly bent. Maintain the elbows at sides and straighten and bend the elbows. Maintain a slight arch in the back and slight bend at the knees.

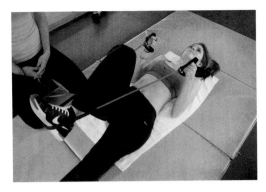
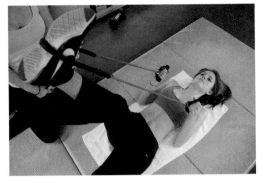

Hamstring Stretch with Band: Place an elastic band around the pad of one foot and lie down flat on the mat. Straighten the free leg and anchor it to the ground. Gently pull the knee of the banded leg into your chest and then slowly extend your knee to a straight leg. Continue to bend and straighten the knee to stretch the hamstring.

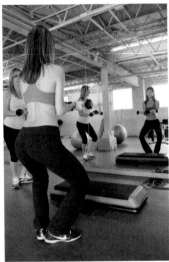
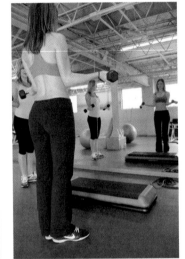

First Position Ballet Squat with External Rotation: Stand in a first position ballet squat. Tuck your hips underneath you and hold 5-pound dumbbells, elbows at a 45-degree angle. As you lower your butt into a squat, externally rotate your arms out to your sides. Your elbows should maintain contact with your ribs. As you return to a standing position, internally rotate your arms back in front of you. Maintain a lifted chest and neutral chin position of your head.

Single Leg Step-Up with Dumbbell: Standing in front of your step, hold a dumbbell in each hand. Place a foot fully on the step and using the leg and gluteus muscle, step-up fully to a standing position. Use the same foot you stepped-up with to return you to the starting position. Repeat with each leg at least fifteen times.

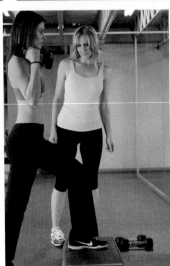
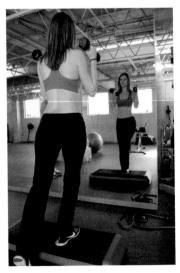
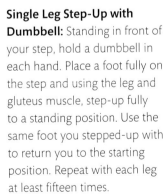

RESISTANCE TRAINING

You can substitute hand weights with resistance bands—those long rubber tubes with handles on each end—for a better burn. In resistance exercises, each effort is performed against a specific opposing force generated by resistance—resistance to being pushed, squeezed, stretched, or bent. Whether pulling or pushing the band, as you stretch the rubber during your repetition, the band is evenly resisting your motion, and resisting all motions up and down, beginning to end, until the exercise is finished.

One of the most important traits to this workout is that it's convenient, in terms of time, money, and even space. A convenient workout is one you're more likely to do and great it's for travel. Let's discuss some more workout techniques, philosophies, and options.

EveryGirl Extra-Credit Tip: Even a little is a lot. There were times I couldn't do all three cycles of the workout, so I would just do two. But at least I did that. Do something little as opposed to nothing.

Joining a Gym

I'm not crazy about gyms. Other gym-goers make going to the gym either a fashion show or a competition. I don't have time for either. Plus, I run like a goof. I'd rather not have that on display.

I'd like to see you avoid joining a gym. They're expensive and crowded, which means time spent waiting for machines and weights. Commuting to the gym consumes precious time, too. We have enough obstacles to keep us from working out, and we don't need to create any more for ourselves. On the flip side, gyms located near work can be ideal. If you do want to opt for a gym membership, do your research. Visit the gym at the hour you think you'll be using it. If it's crowded, you may want to avoid joining. Or you may want to consider gyms that enroll only women.

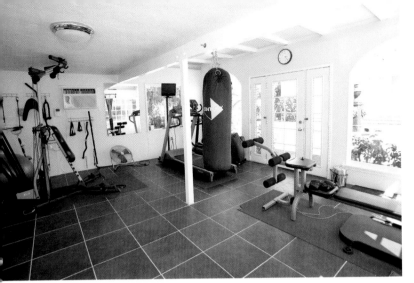

This was an open cabana that we closed and made into a gym.

Home Gym

For the girl who is trying to cram everything into her life, I thoroughly recommend working out at home. The convenience can't be beat. Between the methods of working out today and the amount of equipment on the market, you don't need a great deal of space or money to exercise at home—a few square feet next to your bed is plenty.

My Gym

These days, my house has a separate space for the gym, but you don't need one. In my apartment and in my old house, my home gym was located in my bedroom. I had a treadmill, within viewing distance of my TV, and resistance bands and free weights that I stored neatly under my bed. I tucked my feet under my dresser to do sit-ups, and I got amazing results.

EveryGirl Extra-Credit Tip: Working out in front of your TV and DVR is a great way to catch up on shows.

EveryGirl Extra-Credit Tip: People are always buying exercise stuff that just collects dust. Go to eBay or Craigslist and you'll find great deals on used equipment.

Workout Equipment

What equipment you choose all depends on what you can afford and what space you have. Resistance bands, a few dumbbells, and a four-by-four-foot space is enough.

For Cardio

Cardio is the most important exercise, in my opinion. It's best for keeping weight off, destressing, and getting a good sweat. Running on hard pavement is tough on the legs, though. The bounce of a treadmill is softer and puts less pressure on joints, and with an elliptical machine, you don't really have that pressure at all. I also love the fact that I can watch an episode of *South Park* or *Dateline* while running, using either the elliptical or the treadmill.

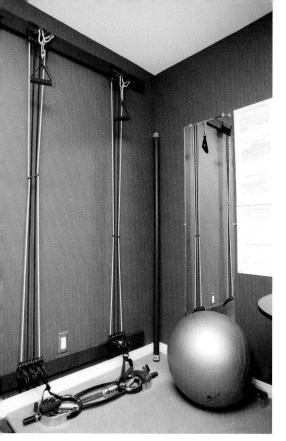

This is a four-by-four-foot space with a long mirror and the Altus Resistance Bands.

For Resistance

I have a Bowflex unit, which I've had for seven years. Bowflex is the best way to get cut and is affordable resistance training that my dad and Keven use, too. If you have a little extra space, a few extra bucks, and guys in your house, Bowflex is a great investment.

A door gym, a great unit for resistance workouts, is hidden conveniently behind a door. The exercises you can do on the Weider X-Factor home gym are similar to the ones you do on the Bowflex. It fits easily to the back of doors with no drilling and sells for under a hundred dollars. The Altus Athletic home gym goes for less than forty. In my production office, I have one of these, which the guys use, too.

Other Pieces

Be open to trying new exercises and new equipment. You get better results when you switch up workout routines. Mats, balls, punching bags, and jump ropes are all great additional pieces to have.

Work Out to Videos

If you don't have the money or space for a treadmill, get your cardio in through a video. It's a great way to get a burn. My favorite video is Harley Pasternak's *5-Factor Fitness* Program. It's only twenty-five minutes—before you know it, you're done.

EveryGirl Extra-Credit Tip: Do some quick exercises before your next big event! I do. When I'm going to be sleeveless or expose my calves at big events like the Oscars or Emmys, I'll do a few quick exercises just before or after I get dressed. I'll do calf raises using a set of stairs and work my arms with resistance bands. I don't work up a sweat, but I do give my muscles a jolt that tightens them up and improves their look for the evening. Just before my debut in the WWE, where I appeared as a guest on Monday night *Raw*, I did sit-ups to get my abs tight. Do the same for big events of your own!

Other Workouts

The Travel Workout

I travel so much. When I don't have room to pack my resistance bands or door gym, I've developed an in-room workout that requires little.

- I do triceps push-ups off a desk, bureau, or bathroom sink.
- I do push-ups off the wall or bureau.
- In bed, with my feet under the covers, I do leg lifts and side leg lifts, too. The blankets create weight and resistance, so it's not easy. I did this one watching the vice presidential debate between Sarah Palin and Joe Biden.
- I even do push-ups and sit-ups on the bed, too. The key is to squeeze everything really tight so you get the most out of the moves. It's a rare way to work out, while in bed!
- My other favorite thing to do in bed is stretching. Every night I will stretch before I fully lie down. I even do a little yoga.
- Lunges and squats also can be done in your room.
- I'll take a big bottle of water and do some biceps curls with it.
- In the car, I will do butt squeezes at stoplights.

EveryGirl Extra-Credit Tip: In the airport, don't use the people movers or escalators. Make a conscious choice to walk the distance and get in extra cardio. As a frequent flyer, I know those are some long, long walks. Take the stairs, too!

These cables are cheap, easy to carry in your suitcase, and very versatile. You can workout every part of your body!

Sumo Squat

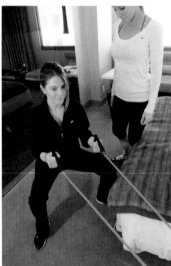

Reverse Lunge with Row

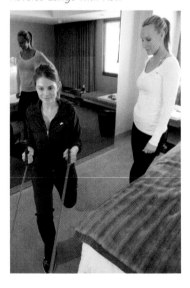

Standing Biceps Curls: Standing with your feet shoulder width apart, stand on a resistance band with both feet to generate tension, and grip the handles with your palms facing forward, elbows at your sides. Keeping your posture tall and shoulders drawn back, pull the palms up toward the shoulders. Stand with a wider grip to create more resistance in the band.

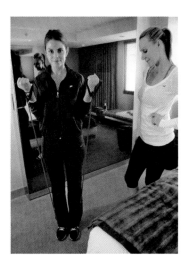

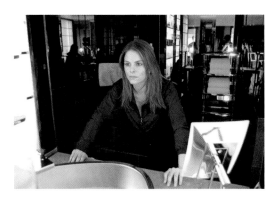

Ledge Push-ups: Find a counter and stand with your feet and hands shoulder width apart. Place your hands on the edge and, using slow and controlled form, lower your straight body toward the counter. With a breath and contracted abs, push away from the counter to the start position.

My Lazy Woman's Workout

I admit to being too lazy for official workouts sometimes. I just find other ways to incorporate working out into my day. Taking the stairs at every turn is the obvious option. On set, I'll randomly do calf raises. In the shower, I'll do the same—just be careful not to slip when you do. I'll do squats in the shower, too.

While cooking, when waiting for something to boil or simmer, I'll do some squats or triceps pushes off the counter. I just find ways to include working out in my daily duties.

When I showed my Lazy Woman's Workout to my trainer Andrea, she said she thought it was brilliant! I was nervous to show her at first. It's not going to yield the same results as a real workout would, but it will do something. And when I don't want to travel with workout gear, it enables me to get something done!

EveryGirl Extra-Credit Tip: Hit the local mall for your cardio—especially during hot or cold weather. I'm seeing more people power walking around mall perimeters. I see packs of moms in full workout attire, quickly pushing baby carriages in unison to tunes from their iPods. And by the way—what a great way to see all the new styles and fashions!

My Lazy Woman's Workout

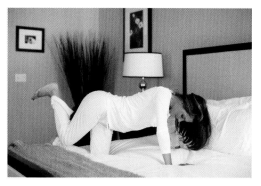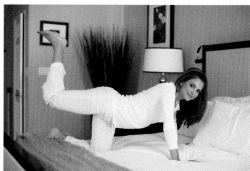

Leg Lifts: Do two sets of twenty, please.

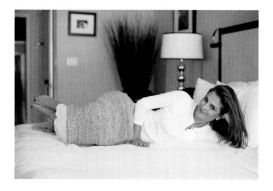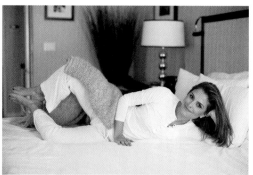

Lateral Clams: The blanket is to add weight and tension. Keep your ankles together and in the air. Slowly lift your leg and keep your ankles close together. Do two sets of twenty.

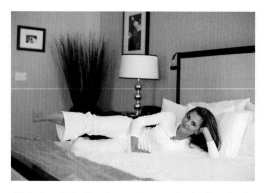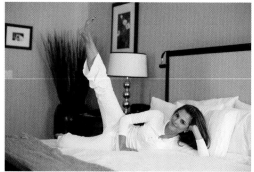

Side Leg Lift: Bend your leg on the bed at the knee. Take your other leg and lift up and down, making sure your ankle crosses over your stationary knee. Do two sets of twenty.

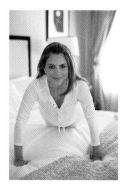
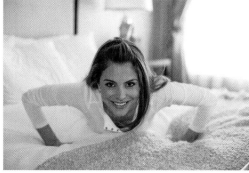

Girly Push-ups: Bend your knees on the bed and then lift and lower your upper body. Do as many as you can.

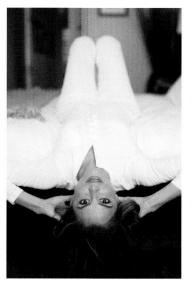

Bed Sit-ups: *(left)* Lie on your back with your shoulders hanging off the edge of the bed. Place your hands behind your head and slowly lift and lower your upper body while squeezing your abs.

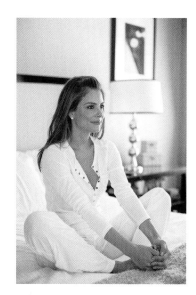

Cobbler's Pose: *(right)* Bring the soles of your feet together and as close to your groin as you can. Press your knees down toward the bed. Hold for twenty seconds or longer.

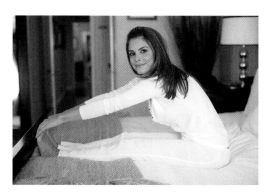
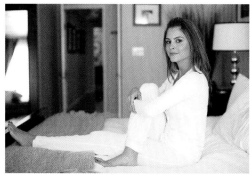

I love to stretch! Hold each stretching pose for twenty seconds or longer.

Cross your leg over the other, hugging it to your body. Repeat on the other leg. Hold for twenty seconds or longer.

The Office Workout

My former executive producer at *Entertainment Tonight*, Linda Bell Blue, lived and breathed the show. But she was human and had to stay healthy like the rest of us, so she had a treadmill in her office and would multitask and get her workout in while at work.

- Maybe you can't have a treadmill in your office, but the bands and dumbbells fit under your desk.
- If you get an hour for lunch, take a half hour to exercise.
- If you have to have a meeting, try doing it over a walk instead of over lunch or coffee. I do it all the time. It makes for great exercise and a more productive meeting.

The Yoga Workout

Many swear by yoga—I'm a new convert. A yogi named Cameron, whom I met at the *Today* show, taught me some poses to help me with my asthma. The most important thing Cameron and yoga taught me, though, is how to breathe correctly—this is something few of us do properly, which causes all sorts of health problems. I now use my inhalers less and have more energy. Yoga will help you to breathe better, too. As far as remaining toned and conditioned, celebrities like Madonna swear by it. I do yoga in the morning—as little or as much as time will permit. It's a great way to start the day.

EveryGirl Extra-Credit Tip: Inhale and exhale—take deep breaths as you inhale and push out your stomach. On the exhale, the stomach should retract. This is proper breathing. Inhaling and exhaling deeply is healthy and will make you feel better. Doing it in the fresh air is even better. If there is a scent you enjoy, like that of a fresh flower or a piece of fruit, then take the time to breathe in deeply and enjoy the aroma.

Yogi Cameron and I are doing yoga stretches. Through controlled breathing and movements I get relaxed and toned.

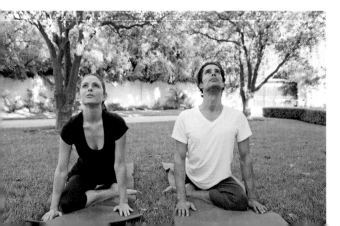
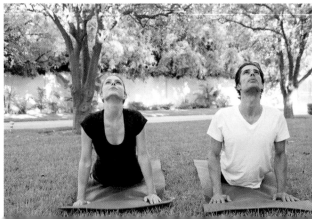

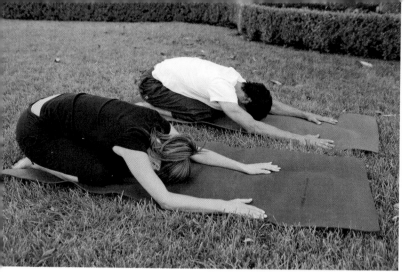

Cameron and I are in child's pose

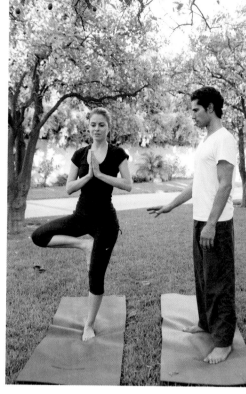

Cameron guides me through a pose.

The Self-Defense Workout

I wanted to travel to Iraq for NBC to do a report on the women there. Knowing how dangerous the environment is, I took Krav Maga classes. Krav Maga is a form of self-defense that ended up giving me more confidence in life, but it was also a fantastic workout, too. It is definitely a creative option.

At the SLS Hotel opening, I was in a full-length gown when I told LA Mayor Antonio Villaraigosa to put an imaginary gun to my back. He did, and I went into action to disarm him—probably a little too much action. He just walked away, stunned. I've since seen his associates, who always laugh about that moment and say, "Maria, the mayor is frightened of you!"

When It Is Time to Relax

Massages

- If you get a good masseur at a spa, ask them if they do house calls. Many like the opportunity for side work. It's more private and convenient and maybe less money, too.
- If you're going to spring for a massage, consider getting a Thai massage, which incorporates stretching.
- When you are shopping at the mall, be sure to hit the gadget stores

that have all the electric massage chairs and devices. Take a load off, sit in the chairs, and get yourself a quick free massage.

- Brookstone has amazing Tempur-Pedic Comfort-Step Slippers. When you come home from work, after a long day in heels, there's no better relief for your feet than slipping a pair on.
- Rolling a kitchen rolling pin over sore muscles is an excellent way to give yourself or someone else a massage. I have Mom and Dad doing it to each other at the end of every day.
- If you don't have a whirlpool, take a good hot bath after a workout or to end your day. Bed Bath & Beyond has great items—like bath pillows, candles, and salts—to make it a rejuvenating spa experience.

Stretch

As we get older, our muscles stiffen and we lose range of motion. Bending and daily activities become harder. Even though my dad has great natural muscle tone, he is definitely stiff and less mobile. Trainer friends have attributed this to his lack of stretching.

A routine stretching program feels good, relieves pains, and lengthens muscles, keeping them spry and youthful. In addition, stretching is believed to reduce the chance of injuries, as well as increase circulation and energy levels. Stretch daily if you can—while you watch TV, sit at your desk, or prepare dinner.

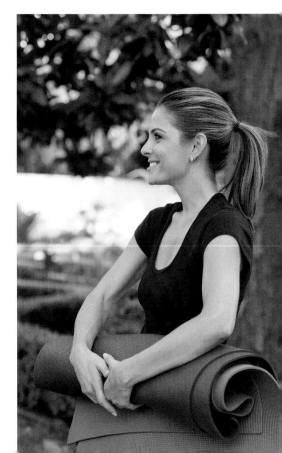

Hire someone reputable to stretch you and teach you stretches you can do alone. Or have them stretch you and your partner and teach you how to stretch each other.

In a small bowl, whisk together the dressing ingredients.

In a separate bowl, mix together the lettuce, tomatoes, onion, and feta cheese.

Fill the pita pocket with the mixture and top with the dressing.

STUFFED ARTICHOKES

Serves 2

4 whole artichokes, stemmed, chokes removed
¼ cup olive oil
3 large yellow onions, sliced
3 cloves garlic, minced
½ cup fresh chopped parsley
Salt and pepper, to taste

Preheat the oven to 300°F.

Fill a pot with an inch of water and add a steamer basket or colander. Place the artichokes in the pot and cover. Over medium heat, steam the artichokes for 5 to 7 minutes, or until tender. Remove from heat.

Heat the olive oil in a saucepan over low heat. Add the onion, garlic, salt, pepper, and parsley, and sauté until golden brown and caramelized.

Coat a baking pan with nonstick cooking spray and arrange the artichokes in the pan. Brush the artichokes with olive oil and season with salt and pepper. Spoon a quarter of the onion mixture into each artichoke and bake for 30 minutes.

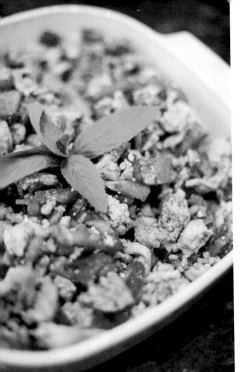

You can eat this in a pita or serve in a dish for a carb-free option.

TURKEY-FETA WRAP

Serves 4

1 pound Jennie-O ground turkey
1 large tomato, chopped
1 medium red onion, chopped
1 cup crumbled low-fat or fat-free feta
Balsamic vinaigrette to taste
4 whole-wheat pita pockets

Coat a pan with nonstick cooking spray. Over medium heat, cook the ground turkey for 2 to 5 minutes, or until all turkey is brown and cooked. Remove from heat and drain.

In a mixing bowl, combine the turkey with the tomato, red onion, and feta. Add the balsamic vinaigrette and toss to coat. Lightly toast the pita and stuff with the turkey mixture.

MARIA'S MUST-HAVE CHOCOLATE FANTASY . . . WITHOUT THE GUILT!

Serves 6

Two 23-gram bags Nabisco Oreo Thin Crisps
Two 1-ounce boxes Jell-O instant sugar-free, fat-free chocolate pudding
1 can sugar-free, fat-free whipped cream
1 39-gram sugar-free Heath bar, crumbled (optional)

Using your hands or a mallet, crush the Oreos in a Ziploc bag.

Follow the instructions to prepare the instant pudding.

Create a small layer of the crushed cookies at the bottom of a wineglass. Then add some pudding.

Layer more crushed cookies, then the whipped cream. Add more pudding. Keep alternating layers as much as you like. I usually do one or two layers each of whipped cream and cookie.

Top off the glass with more crushed Oreo and Heath bar, if you choose. Repeat to fill wineglasses.

Place them in the fridge until you are ready to serve. Top with whipped cream.

THE EveryGirl Kitchen: Maria's Must-Haves

- A Magic Bullet to make protein shakes, salad dressings, and just about anything else! Just add powder and milk and go!
- A measurement conversion chart! I never paid attention in high school to that stuff, and now I wish I had because portions do matter—a lot.

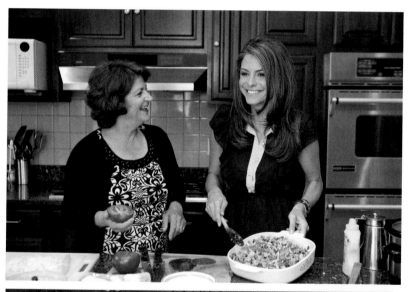

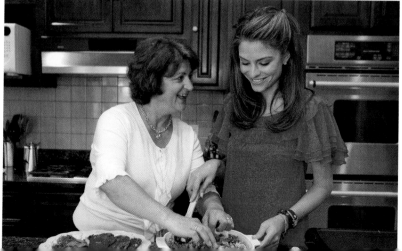

EveryGirl Health and Well-Being

Your health is vital, and *nothing* can be enjoyed if it is compromised.

Find a doctor who won't rush you out and who won't roll his or her eyes when you ask questions or when you initiate alternative ideas for healing; find one who *will* take the time to listen to you and be sensitive to your needs. Sadly, even the good doctors today are so busy with their overwhelming roster of patients that it's easy not to get the most accurate diagnosis and most attentive treatment.

Therefore, you must be as much your own doctor as your doctor is. Living in the age of the Internet, there is helpful information out there on ailments, medicines, and treatments. Pay close attention to the signals your body is sending (pain, tiredness, numbness, lumps, and bumps), and then combine the best information from your doctor with research you can do on your own. An informed patient is one who makes smart choices.

A MARIA MOMENT

A medical emergency occurred with my standard poodle, Athena.

I know Athena's not human, but work with me. Her stomach was distended, and she was gagging. Keven took her to the hospital while I typed the symptoms into an online search engine. Within two minutes, I learned it was gastric dilatation, or bloat. I texted the info to Keven, which helped expedite her treatment and save her life.

EveryGirl Medical Tips

- If you can't afford health insurance, then look into low-cost policies with large deductibles. You may not get treatment for small injuries or ailments, but you'll have insurance that will cover the big emergencies, such as an accident or horrible disease.

- Keep a running list, in your BlackBerry or in a notebook, of symptoms, pains, and ailments you would like to discuss with your doctor. I used to forget and thus prevented myself from getting the best diagnosis or treatment.

- For more serious illnesses and afflictions, have someone accompany you to doctors' visits, like a parent, sibling, BF, or partner. They'll remember to ask questions you won't and help calm your fears.

- Become familiar with your family medical history. You'll learn what you're prone to and may be able to apply precautionary measures.

- Always ask doctors about the side effects of medicines and be sure to double-check online.

- Read up on alternative medicine. We have become so accustomed to wanting the quick-fix pills. There are many natural cures for ailments, like castor oil, tea tree oil, and coconut oil. All of these have helped me; it just takes a little research.

HEALING COLDS

Attack colds! If you don't, they linger and seriously inhibit your quality of life. Take zinc (Zicam is great for colds; Cold-EEZE is great for sore throats) and drink lots of fluids and get lots of sleep. When I feel myself getting sick, I buy Jamba Juices with Immunity Boosts. Sleep is the best medicine for colds. You can also sweat colds out through steam baths. You can turn your shower into a steam bath by running hot water and closing the doors.

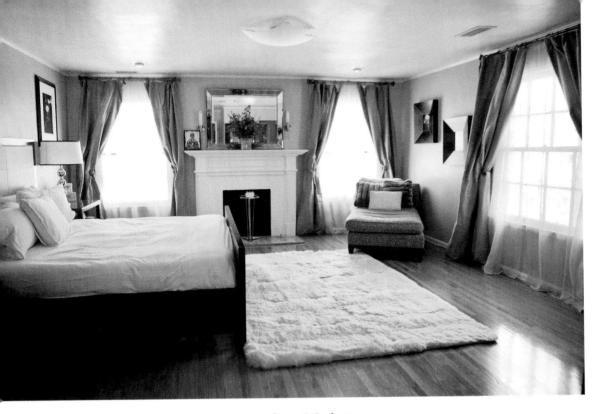

I used calming neutral colors in my bedroom. It's a place for me to relax and catch up on much- needed rest.

Preventative Maintenance

The best defense is a great offense—the same goes when it comes to your health. You need to get yourself as healthy as possible to avoid getting sick in the first place.

Take Your Vitamins

I hate taking vitamins. I believe if you eat well, you should be getting enough nutrients from your food. I hate the smell of them as well as the chore of swallowing them. The vitamins I like are called Yummi Bears Organics. They are chewable and taste like sour gummies.

Get Good Sleep

Good sleep doesn't just cure colds; it speeds up healing of injuries and other illnesses. It also improves your health. Experts believe you need seven to nine hours of unin-

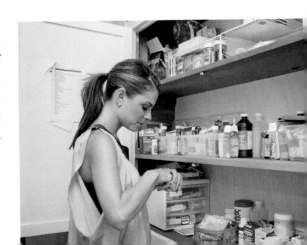

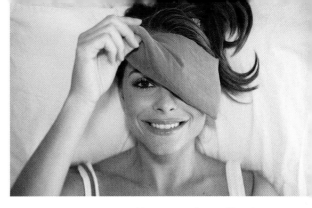

terrupted sleep each night. You'll be more energetic and alert, and you'll age better, too.

They don't call it beauty sleep for nothing! When you sleep, your skin repairs itself and rejuvenates its youthful glow. Have you ever seen young stars who party all night long? They age ten years in the blink of an eye from a lack of sleep.

I love scented eye pillows! They put me right to sleep.

The Momma Bear's Bed . . .

Your bed, and the quality of the mattress you sleep on, are an important part of your foundation. You spend up to one-third of your life in bed, and sleep is just about the best natural form of medicine around. Invest the time and money into getting a mattress that will give you the best night's sleep possible. If you do your research, you can find one that's affordable and right for you. Keep in mind it's a long-term investment.

How to Get Quality Zs

- Don't leave your phone or BlackBerry by your bed. If you do, shut off the ringer.
- A cold, dark room makes for the best sleep environment. Invest in good sheets and a nice comforter.
- Wind down before you go to bed with tea, a walk, or a warm bath. Don't do stimulating activities, like exercise or watching movies or TV shows, right before bed. Also, stop drinking caffeine three hours before bedtime.
- Working in bed is proven to hurt sleep patterns. The nights I do, I definitely don't get the deepest sleep.
- Run a small fan. The hum will drown out any other noise and lull you to sleep. You could try a sound machine, too.
- If you go to bed listening to the radio or watching TV, then I recommend a sleep timer that will force the radio or TV to go off after an hour or so. If the radio or TV stays on, your mind will still be working, in a sense, depriving you of deep sleep. You'll feel less rested the next day.

EveryGirl Mental Health Is Just as Important

When you are stressed or upset, you are greatly increasing your chances of getting sick. You need to find cost- and time-effective ways to ease tension, such as exercising, getting a massage, stretching, yoga, taking baths, and having fun. My friend, psychologist Dr. Gia Marson, emphasizes the importance of staying in the moment while you're doing your stress-busting activity.

"I take a bath every night and light a candle. It's the time I relax. I bring my phone and a glass of wine. It's my time."

—Shelley Zalis, founder and CEO of OTX

Meditate

Jerry Seinfeld, Russell Simmons, and Howard Stern are just a few who practice, and credit success to, meditation. The purpose behind meditation is for your mind to move beyond thinking and into a deeper state of relaxation and awareness. Meditation is as simple as listening to, and focusing on, anything from singing birds to brushing your dogs to listening to your own breathing, all with your mind free from any other distractions.

During meditation, you can focus, daydream, and visualize what you want in life, from the kind of house you'll live in to the career you want. Most of what I've visualized and hoped for has come true.

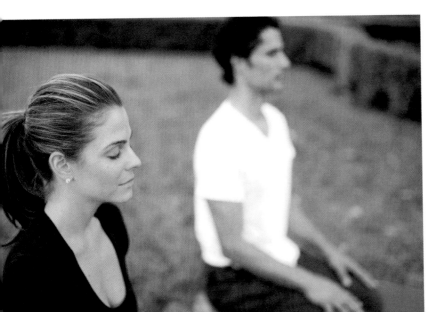

I'm in the process of learning more about meditation. There are meditation centers where you can learn more, too. But at the end of the day, it's just about taking fifteen minutes to relax, breathe deeply, and focus your mind on one thing.

Reiki

Reiki is a Japanese technique and form of meditation and energy healing used for stress reduction and healing. We used Reiki on one of our sick dogs. We allotted time each night to do so, just holding her close and focusing on one thing: her healing. It really made a difference. You can practice Reiki on others and yourself, too, and learn more about it online.

Benefits of Meditation

- It relaxes muscles and reduces tension, which in turn, can relieve headaches and migraines, high blood pressure, and other stress-related ailments and can even help with premenstrual syndrome.
- It boosts your immune system and can help you heal and recover more quickly. There are umpteen stories of people who have beat cancer through meditation.
- It improves your mental strength and ability to concentrate.
- It increases serotonin levels in your brain. Low levels of serotonin are associated with depression, obesity, insomnia, and headaches.
- It helps you to cope with phobias and deep-seated inner pains and issues that take a toll on your mental, as well as your physical, health.
- It puts mothers more deeply in tune with their babies—before and after they're born.
- It helps you achieve tasks and goals.

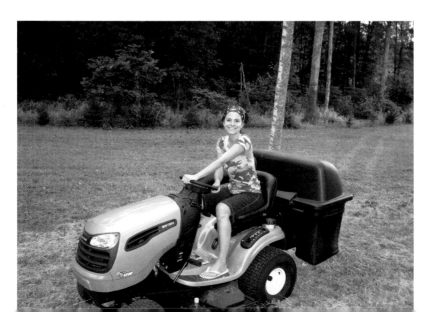

When I'm home in Connecticut, one of the ways I relax is by mowing the lawn. The smell of the grass and the activity helps clear my head.

EveryGirl Gets the Blues

We all get the blues now and again. But I asked friend, psychologist, and EveryGirl Expert Dr. Gia Marson for ways we can identify when a case of the blues in ourselves or our friends might be a bit more serious, and how to help a friend in need.

Q: How does EveryGirl know when she needs to get a little bit of professional help?

A: Let's assume you know there is a problem and are trying to decide how serious it is. Check three areas to decide if your girlfriend needs professional help.

1. What is the *duration* of the problem? Does it seem as if the distress has gone on too long? Trust your instincts. If your friend does not seem to be adjusting over time to a life event or transition, she may need some help to do so.
2. What is the *intensity* of the problem? Does her reaction seem to be about what you might expect? If she has any suicidal thoughts, she definitely needs professional help.
3. What amount of *interference* is her problem causing? Is she risking something important because she is not coping well? If whatever ails her is causing such a decline in functioning that it is risking her health, relationships, or work, it may also be time for professional help.

If you decide to talk to her about it, here are some guidelines. Tell her what you are observing without making any assumptions about what your observations mean, offer to support her in getting help, and have resources ready. Just a thought . . . I don't believe professional help is only for those who need it. Many girls come to professionals to improve on their already high-functioning selves. *Kaizen* is all about continuous improvement. If things are good in your life, therapy may make them even better!

Q: How can you pull yourself out of the blues?

A: Obviously, life can be very hard at times. But while the blues are a normal part of life, there are ways you can simultaneously acknowledge the experience (remember no avoiding negative feelings) and take steps to feel better. To pull yourself out of the blues, connect with others and notice what you are grateful for. The old adage that "time heals all wounds" is true as well. So, use distraction as a way to cope until time passes. Remember in difficult times to focus on the basics by being especially conscientious about eating well, getting enough sleep, being active, and reaching out for support.

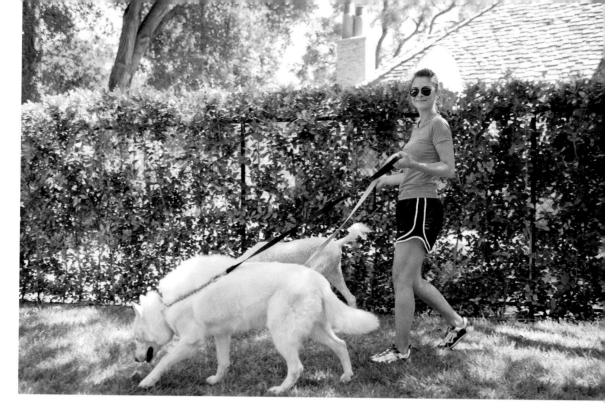

Beating the Blues

- To help beat depression, keep your mind and your hands as active and as occupied as possible.
- Try something new if you have the blues. Try a new hairstyle or a new style altogether. A little change can have a big impact.
- Crank the tunes. I love driving, working out, and getting ready with great music playing. It always lifts my spirits. Sing out loud, too. It's a great release.
- Clean and reorganize your house. It will keep you busy and you'll feel better after you do.

Clean Up Your Act

I've seen depressed people let themselves go in a big way. They've gained weight, let their homes fall apart, and stopped caring for, and about, themselves. If you're engaging in this kind of behavior (or know a friend who is), put a halt to it. I know this is just a start to healing a major problem, but it should be the first step.

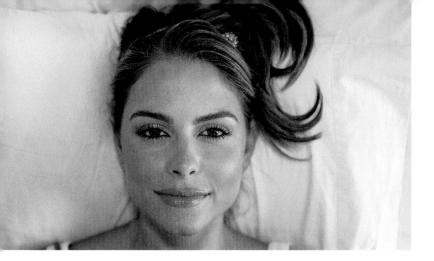

Talk out problems with others who might be able to help you make a fresh start.

Talk It Out

Keep talking to people who will listen *and* be a good listener to someone else who's depressed. Purging is the best way to heal. Talking to a professional therapist is great, too. If you can't afford one, then look online for free services and support groups. There are lots out there.

Coping with Loss

Sixteen years later I am still crushed over the untimely death of my eighteen-year-old cousin Narge. I also know people who have been devastated by breakups or divorce. Loss is brutal and something I struggle with. With time, you will heal, no matter how hopeless it may seem. In the meantime, keep busy, try new things, and talk it out.

And whatever you do, don't give up . . . please. Work to heal yourself and reach out for help.

EveryGirl Extra-Credit Tip: If you're experiencing heartache or having a minor anxiety attack (and it's not serious), pick up a hot-water bottle at the local pharmacy. Fill with hot water, wrap it in a towel, and place it on your chest. The weight and the warmth of the bottle will soothe and calm you.

Give and You Shall Receive

Working with those in need—whether they be animals or people—helps distract you from your own woes, reminds you of those who have it worse, and empowers you in knowing you were able to help someone else.

Here I am with my cousin Narge and my other cousins. I miss Narge dearly and love him.

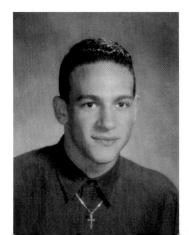

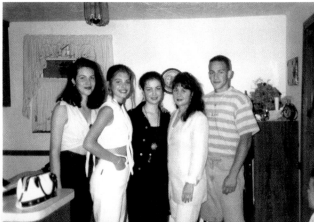

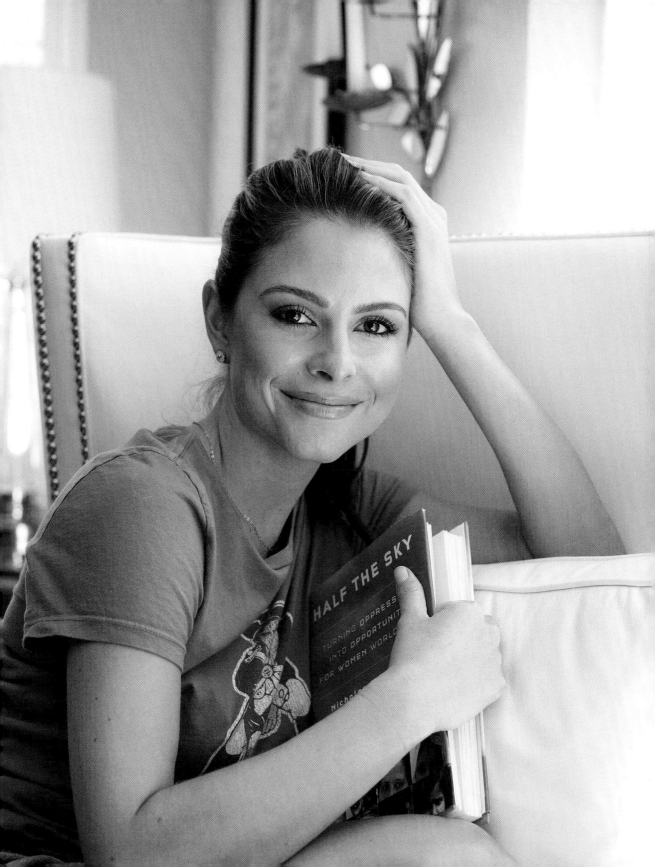

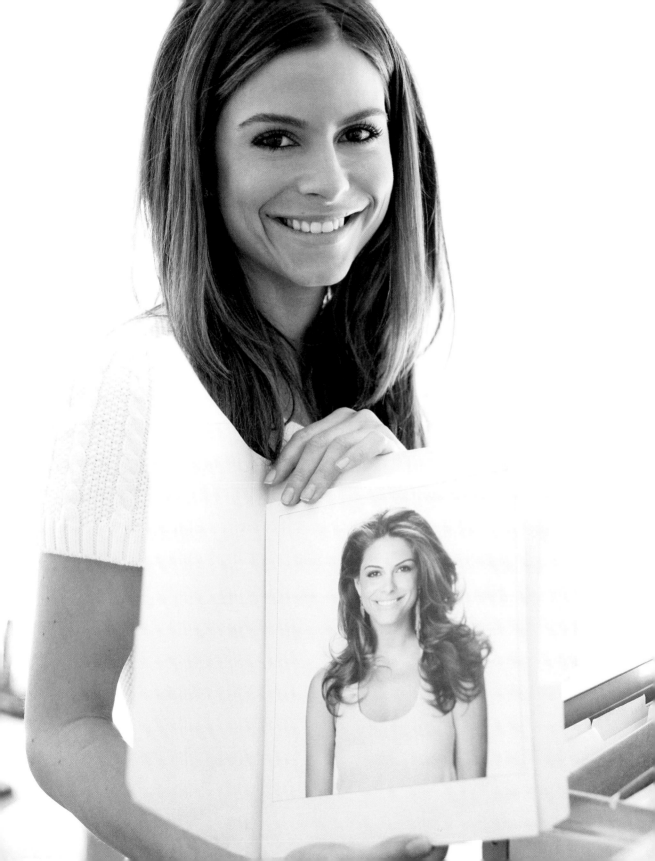

part five

EveryGirl
Business

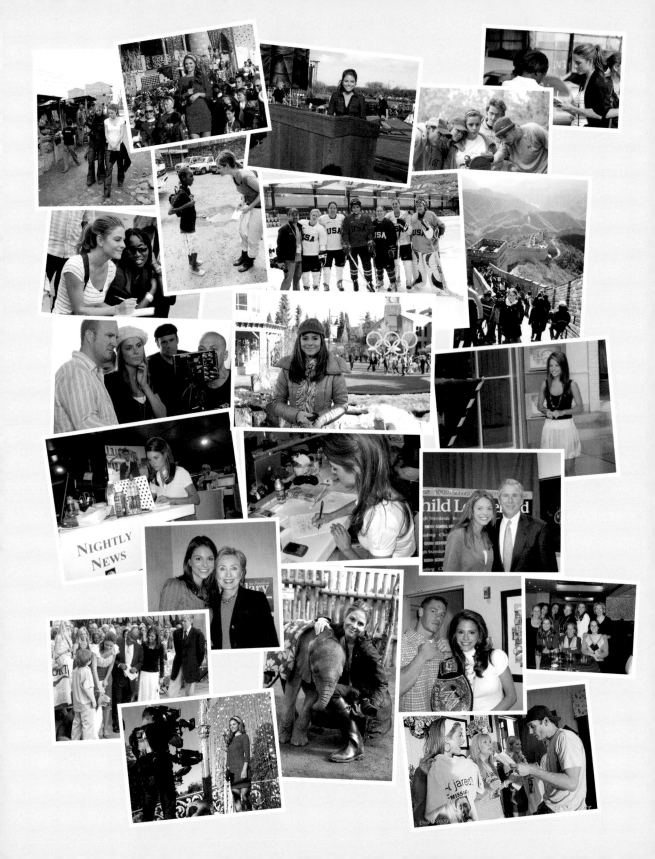

WHETHER YOU'RE GOING TO BE A STAY-AT-HOME MOM OR A WORKING MOM OR JUST A WORKING WOMAN, YOU NEED TO KNOW A FEW THINGS ABOUT BUSINESS. Being business-savvy while at home is just as important as it is at the office. It will help you run your household and set a great example for your children, too. Also, should you sadly be forced to survive the loss of a partner, you'll be better prepared to pick up the pieces.

How to work, how to negotiate, how to get ahead, and how to manage others are just a few of the many things that you need to learn, not only for business but for all aspects of your life. It's all part of EveryGirl's business.

EveryGirl Rules to Live By

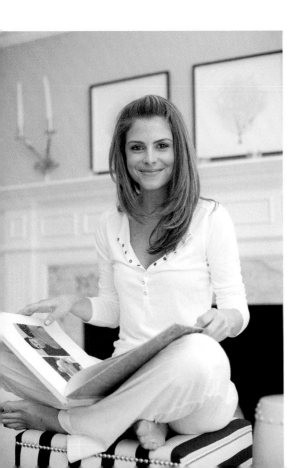

Among my hopes for this book are that I will help you to organize and clean your homes, teach you how to do your hair and makeup, show you how to exercise and how to dress, and encourage you to make healthy life choices. Overall, I hope to help you build a good foundation for your life, but in the end, it is your job to keep the foundation strong and build your own house.

To do this, you must have the right attitude, the right mind-set, and the proper knowledge of how to handle everyday life situations. The following are mottos and morals I've learned thus far that have helped me build a strong foundation for my own life.

EveryGirl *Doesn't* Believe in Santa

Santa's going to give us that pay raise. Santa's going to get us that promotion. Santa's going to find us that perfect companion. Santa's going to bring us everything we want or need in life. And when Santa doesn't bring us what we want—because he doesn't exist—we usually feel helpless, hurt, angry, bitter, resentful, depressed, or some combination of the above.

I know I always believed in Santa. My parents did,

too. We thought bosses, accountants, doctors, and every other professional, including hairdressers for that matter, knew better and would always give us exactly what we needed or deserved.

People in my own industry believe Santa came to me. They think I got lucky. What they don't know is that when I got my job at *Entertainment Tonight*, the first thing I did was hire a publicist. At the time, no other broadcast journalist had really ever had one. Among other sacrifices, I lived in a rough neighborhood to even afford one, but it got me publicity, which led to all the opportunities in acting and commercials.

The success you have and the things you achieve will not be luck or gifts from Santa. They will come from your hard work and wise choices, and from being proactive.

Do Micromanage

So many celebrities will look at more successful celebrities and say, "They *must* have the best managers." *Wrong.* The most successful celebs *are* their own best managers! Do you really think that Oprah's managers and agents made her? Oprah has an overall vision for her life that she has executed to perfection. You can do the same.

It's about the small stuff: taking magazine cutouts to hairdressers to show them the style you want and taking nondesigner clothes to the tailor to custom-create designs for yourself. It's about the bigger stuff:

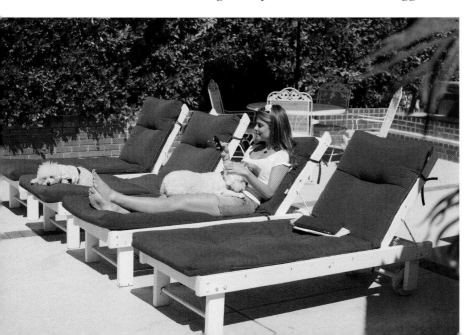

As long as I have my PDA and remain organized, I can manage my work and life from just about anywhere.

researching tax laws online and bringing your findings to your accountant, and using the Internet and medical journals to help doctors treat you.

It's about managing your managers and knowing "expert" is not another word for God.

But Also Listen . . .

When managers or your advisory committee advise you—whether you agree or not—listen! Hear them out. Many have already made the mistakes for you. I see people in my business continually ignore amazing advice, then wonder why they never get ahead. Listen to the genuine advice of others with more experience. There will be times to override their advice—you know you hold final veto—but maybe not as often as you might think.

The Story of Noelle

One day my apricot rescue poodle, Noelle, stopped walking. One vet wanted thousands just to run tests, and another gave her two months to live. If I believed in Santa, I would have waited for a miracle or listened to the vets who wanted to put her to sleep. Instead we researched her condition, chatted with other pet lovers, and got her supplements. For Noelle's legs, Mom sewed padded Velcro cuffs that enabled her to hop. She swam every day, too. In the winter, we put her in the tub, where, attached to a harness, she swam in place. We had five more wonderful years with her after that.

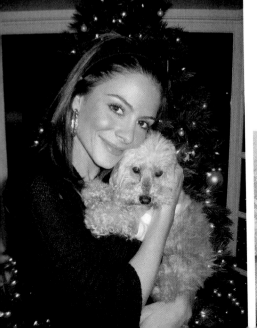

We created a beautiful grave site for Noelle that we visit in our yard. There are many online companies that custom make the stone.

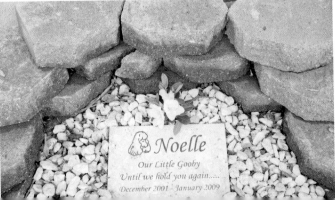

Remember Who Is Paying Whom

You're paying your nanny, doctor, and accountant. My mom and dad were eager to please employers because their employers were paying them. I'm the same way at NBC as I was at Dunkin' Donuts. Yet we're all often bullied by the people we pay. Don't be. Remember who is paying whom.

Hire Pleasers

Successful women hire pleasers in their various support positions. These are the gems of the world who enjoy caring for and pleasing others. I always loved pleasing the people I work for and still do.

By pleaser, I don't mean pushover. Jayne, my dog walker, is a pleaser who enjoys making my life easier. However, she's no pushover. She has no problem standing her ground against me—for what she believes is best for my dogs.

MANAGING STAFF

This box is for the advanced EveryGirl who has household employees to manage, i.e., assistants, nannies, housekeepers, etc.

Though I'm a firm believer in being as independent and hands-on as possible, there are times when you'll need support to be successful. As you know, I wasn't born into my current lifestyle. My parents never had housekeepers or landscapers or assistants or dog walkers. We were those things for other people. But all of our employers loved us because we were honest, hardworking, and eager to please.

With a strong foundation, and your black book, having someone step in to help is much easier. Below are some tips that will help.

- For home assistants, housekeepers, dog walkers, and nannies alike, have them supply you with a daily update of what they accomplished. If they are working on ongoing projects for you—organizing all the family photo albums, for instance—then have them write about the status of the projects. My dog walker, Jayne, actually taught me this. She leaves a note for me every day: BRUSHED APOLLO, PUT MEDICINE IN ATHENA'S EARS, AND TOOK GANG FOR A WALK. She'll also alert me to problems, such as LATCH ON GATE IS BROKEN or HOSE IS LEAKING. Bottom line: the daily update is invaluable for both you and your help.
- Keep a running to-do list for staff in your tasks folder on your PDA to remind you and them. And never assume that once you give them a task it will just get done. It's only when they write that it's been completed on their daily update that you should delete it.

- Issue their first paycheck a week or two after they begin work. Ever wonder why employers do this to you? Withholding a pending check reduces the chance of them running away with the house keys, PDA, or laptop that you may have issued them.
- Switch to more expensive house locks and keys—the kind that cannot be copied without a specific code card. You can also have a coded lockbox on your property—the kind realtors put on house doors. You and the worker will be the only ones with the code, and the house key will always remain on the property. It comes in handy when you're locked out!
- If the person you hire will be e-mailing people for you, then create a password and e-mail account for that person that looks like this: mariaasst@hotmail.com. For the address, use your first name or the name of your company and then attach "asst" (short for assistant) to that name, using whatever e-mail server you can afford—Windows Live Hotmail, Yahoo!, etc. This enables you to keep precious info long after they have left, and your associates will always have the correct info for your most current assistant.
- Hire for heart . . . train for skill. It's often better to hire someone who may be inexperienced but wants to work hard and learn, rather than someone who has the experience and skills but doesn't want to work hard and adapt.

Embrace Research:
Take Advantage of the Internet

The Internet is the most amazing resource for answers on every subject. Put it to good use.

There are a variety of help experts online who will answer your questions for fees as low as fifteen dollars. You can use search engines like Bing to find experts who can troubleshoot problems for you in mechanics, electronics, law, fashion, and everything in between. Justanswer.com is one of many websites that allow you to e-mail such experts. When my treadmill stopped working, I used one such expert, and he saved me hundreds of dollars.

Remember, when using the Internet for research, apply wisdom and a degree of skepticism. Read everyone's opinions and scrutinize the information carefully. Some positive opinions may be lies propagated to sell products, and some could be misinformation.

Make the Universe Your Friend

When it comes to questions, from who the right guy is for you to what job you should take to decisions of all kinds, don't be afraid to ask the universe. Answers to your questions will come in ways you never imagined. Just be aware of her presence and the signs she sends you.

Seek to Create Win-Win Scenarios

Don't be afraid to ask your manicurist, hairdresser, or masseur to come by your house, where it's more convenient for you. Many work for less and will gladly take you up on your offer. As I've said before, "Ask and you shall receive!"

When you get a great manicurist to come to your house to do your nails (for convenience) and pay her a sum greater than the wage her employer is paying, you are creating a win-win scenario. The win-win is the most fun to take part in, and I do it all the time.

At work, I'm constantly thinking of ways for my employers to win along with me, and it's great for both sides.

EveryGirl Extra-Credit Tip: Pick up the best-selling book *The Secret* for more help with making the universe your friend.

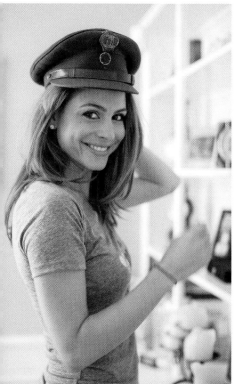

Take command of your world and those you employ. You'd be surprised at how willing others are to follow your lead.

Go Green

A greener lifestyle is good not just for the world: it's good for your wallet. Between hosting the Planet Green show *Hollywood Green with Maria Menounos*, my work with Future Friendly, and being victimized by this dreadful economy, I adapted a greener lifestyle and am so much happier since doing so. A greener lifestyle has saved me time and money, all while doing right by the environment. I am by no means someone who is totally green, mind you. I'm someone who is taking baby steps with it all and trying to explain to others how to do the same.

How I Stay Green

- I own a hybrid car.
- I don't heat or air-condition the whole house and use them sparingly.
- I always shut off the heat and AC before I leave, and I posted a sign reminding all in the house to do the same.
- I turn the heat down each night. Sleeping bundled up in cooler climates yields better sleep, too!
- I reuse towels (just not my faceclothes, ha-ha).
- I use few dishes, washing and drying them by hand.
- I use minimal water on my lawn.
- I launder all clothes in cold water. This saves tons of energy, as 80 to 90 percent goes toward heating the water.
- Rather than throw things out, I spruce them up and reuse them or donate them to charity.
- I have designated containers for empty cans and bottles.
- I have a Pur water filter hooked up to my sink. It provides fresh drinking water and saves me from buying and lugging plastic bottles. I use it to fill a water jug, which I keep at my desk, bedside, and near me during workouts.
- I've also installed a water filter in the bathroom closest to my bedroom so that I have water near my bed, rather than having to trek down to the kitchen for refills.
- I grow my own vegetables.
- I look at the whole green movement as fun, simple, and more cost-effective. It will pay off big for the world and for you.

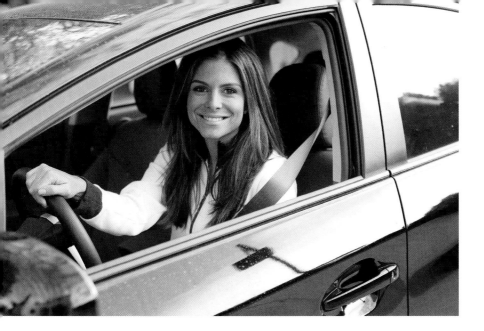

Act, but Don't React

When many of us are mad or hurt, when we feel cheated or even feel bad for others, we "react." Without thinking, we engage in knee-jerk reactions: yelling, throwing tantrums, acting vengefully, saying things we can never take back, or even promising the moon and the stars. All are unhealthy reactions that we'll likely later regret. Some have permanent ramifications. The proper act is to take a moment and really think about the right thing to say and the proper way to respond—considering all potential ramifications. *Responding*, rather than reacting, is replying with a clear head.

> ### A MARIA MOMENT
>
> Friends from home asked to come to LA and stay at my apartment. Without thinking, I agreed. They came in at all hours, kept me from sleeping, and borrowed my car, making me late for work my very first month at *Entertainment Tonight*! If I had taken time to think about it, I would have realized how toxic their visit would be to my future, and I would have politely declined. (On a side note, because I rebuilt my emotional foundation, these "friends" are no longer in my life.)

EveryGirl Extra-Credit Tip: "Let me get back to you." Whether you're offered a salary or asked to babysit for a friend's kids, "Let me get back to you" is the best response. It provides you with ample time to think the situation out clearly so you can later respond properly.

EveryGirl Extra-Credit Tip: We're all good at something, and we all have something to offer. Don't be shy about offering something you can do to get a service you need in return.

How You Can Respond and Not React: A Few Easy Steps

- When you're initially upset, take a beat or longer. Breathe. Curb your emotions and resist reacting irrationally.
- Take as long as you need to think about what you're going to say.
- If reacting has always been a problem and responding is something altogether new, have some reusable stock phrases on hand to allow you time to simmer down and think things through: e.g., *I need a beat to digest this; I don't know how I feel about this;* or *You're catching me off guard—let me have a moment.*
- Question whether you need to defend yourself at all.
- For a moment (even if it's tough), try to see their side of things.
- Think about the long-term consequences of your response.
- Remember how reacting has hurt you in the past; draw from that as inspiration.
- Seek out healthy partners and friends who will help you to see situations more clearly and coach you on how to respond.

The Only Time to Care About What Others Say About You . . .

EveryGirl Extra-Credit Tip: Ask your advisory committee and others you trust for recommendations on plumbers, mechanics, and hairstylists. I found a therapist right down the street from my house through asking friends!

A bunch of female celebs and I were at an event recently, lamenting about how cruel the press and people on the Web can be. An old manager overheard and gave us great advice that I will pass on to you: Care about what people think of you only if your business is predicated on it. If you are running for office or have clients who must like and trust you in order to work with you, then you must care what they say or think. But even then, you can care only so much. There are always going to be people who are jealous, spread gossip, say mean things, and have false perceptions of you. Living your life according to what they think is like blowing into a vacuum. It's an exhausting and pointless way to suffocate. You need to live your life on your own terms.

What We Want vs. What We Really Want

We *want* to marry an amazing guy who will treat us like a queen, but what we *really want* is the hot guy stud who is self-centered and who treat us like crap. We all *want* to live a long and healthy life, but what we *really want* to do is to smoke and drink our heads off. We all *want* to be in shape, but what we *really want* is to eat bad food to excess and not exercise. We all *want* to be wealthy but what we *really want* is to spend all of our hard-earned money on frivolous items and not sacrifice. You get the picture. Figure out what it is that you *want* and then turn it into what you *really want*!

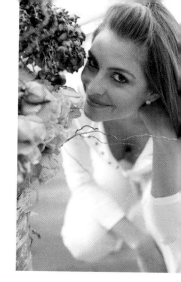

Remember to take a deep breath whenever you feel overwhelmed and stop and smell the flowers!

A Maria Moment: Have Mercy on Yourself

I did a great *Dateline* interview with actor Todd Bridges, who told me you need to have mercy on yourself. You give others a break. Why not give yourself one for the mistakes you've made? Nobody, not even the most successful person in the world, goes through life without making blunders. Mistakes are necessary for us to grow. Own up to yours; the only mistake is not learning from them. But don't forget to have mercy on yourself in the process.

EveryGirl Makes Mistakes

As much as I preach in this book from my EveryGirl success pulpit, please know that I have made, and continue to make, many mistakes. I still unintentionally say inappropriate things. I still react, get hypersensitive, spread myself thin, and allow vampires into my life, too, along with other errors. The only real mistake is to stop trying to learn from them and to stop trying to improve. I try every day. We all should, as long as we are on this earth.

At the end of the day, no matter how many life lessons, rules, or mottos you learn, you're still going to screw up. Just don't let it get you down.

CHAPTER SIXTEEN

EveryGirl at Work

Honestly, a lot of my career success has come from applying the philosophies you've already read about in this book. But maybe writing a little about my own work journey will give you some added reinforcement.

When it has come to my jobs, I have always given a hundred percent and done my best to make them fun, too—starting at the age of three. My parents were janitors for a Boston nightclub called the Channel. They couldn't afford a babysitter and wouldn't have trusted one to watch me even if they could have. As they were immigrants in a new country, who could blame them?

While other families got to sleep late on weekends and have fun, we were up and at work by 5 A.M. We'd open the doors of the club as the exhaust of stale beer, cigarette smoke, and vomit poured out. But we never let it get us down. My dad would sing Greek songs as he worked, and I used to Rollerblade through the club as I mopped the floors—dancing and singing, too. It was great bonding time for the family.

Finding loose change became a game, and any extra money we found was put in an empty propane tank under the bar. That money eventually paid for our family trips to Disney World and Greece! When the Channel shut down, I went to work at Dunkin' Donuts.

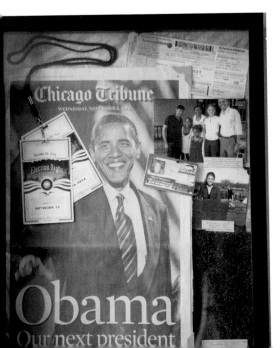

One of the biggest moments in my career: interviewing the Obamas. I framed all the mementos from the campaign.

Some Newsy Events, Topics, and People Covered by Maria

- Barack Obama's presidential run for office. I was on the campaign trail for more than a year and covered both the Republican National Convention and the Democratic National Convention.
- Election-night coverage
- Inauguration coverage
- An AIDS series covered from South Africa
- The 2010 earthquake in El Salvador
- Brush fires in California
- Immigrant kids
- Post-traumatic stress disorder in the military
- Interviews on location with Barack Obama, Michelle Obama, Hillary Clinton, Bill Clinton, George W. Bush, John McCain, John Edwards
- The first family interview with the Obamas

I was there every morning at the crack of dawn. With my paycheck, I could finally buy my own clothes, plus I met so many great people there. I also developed skills there that I employ today.

Let me share a funny Dunkin' Donuts story that speaks directly to my point. I used to watch Vanna White on *Wheel of Fortune* and tell my mom how much I wanted her job. With her Greek accent, my mother used to say, "Maria, her job is ved-dee hard. She has a lot to memorize." I figured if, when taking orders, I could grab the right doughnuts from the racks without looking at the labels, I, too, could one day do Vanna's job. So I worked hard to memorize where all the donuts were. Emulating Vanna's posture and smile, I would wait on customers by picking their doughnuts as Vanna would turn letters on *Wheel of Fortune*. Goofy as it sounds, it was fun. More important, it helped to build my confidence and develop memory skills.

I also memorized regular customers' orders: what kind of doughnut they wanted and how they

On July 4, 2010, Keven accompanied me to Butte, Montana, to interview the Obamas. P.S. They were super down to earth and the kids were as adorable as they appeared.

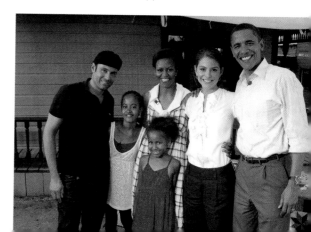

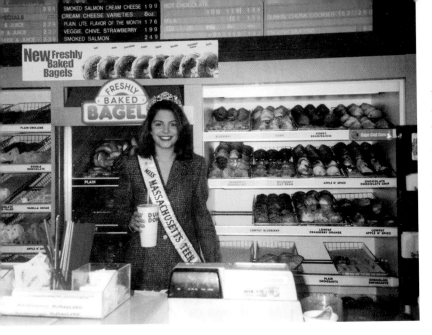

took their coffee. Did I want to sleep in at times? Was I envious of kids who'd come into Dunkin' Donuts on their way to the beach? Of course I was. But making the work fun got me through it all. And you know what else? Working on those weekends and sacrificing as I did instilled a work ethic in me that paid off hugely. Today, I have the most fun of everyone.

One of my first jobs was at Dunkin' Donuts. When I won Miss Massachusetts I made an appearance.

EveryGirl Extra-Credit Tip: Lack the confidence to get onstage and be in a pageant? Find a friend who does and manage her as she competes. By soliciting donors, picking out her gown, assisting her with hair and makeup, and so on, you can gain many of the positive aspects of the experience without the pressure.

I worked in this way at every other job, from perfume spritzer to street sausage vendor, trophy-store clerk to a volunteer on Keven's movie. It was through those contacts that I learned about a job opening at Channel One News, a news program broadcast into classrooms nationwide and, as I said, the place Anderson Cooper got his start.

Remember what I've been saying about having a sense of urgency? As soon as I found out Channel One was looking for new anchors, I went into action—researching everything I could on it. I called Keven and asked him to help me create a reel. (A reel is video highlight footage of you at work, reporting, acting, hosting, etc.) I sent them the reel along with a head shot, resume, and cover letter. In the cover letter, I was sure to express to Channel One everything about myself and how positive, eager, and hardworking I was, as well as my thoughts on the news and the channel. I went into detailed specifics. Sure enough, they called and scheduled an interview in New York. Channel One liked the fact I was diverse in my skills, having produced a movie while learning the news, and I got the job.

As I said, my overprotective Greek father was against me moving to LA, so I was truly on my own family-wise. It was painful and scary, especially from a financial aspect. I just put all that energy into my work at Channel One. *Entertainment Tonight*'s Brad Bessey, and later Linda Bell Blue, saw my work on Channel One, and that led to me getting my true

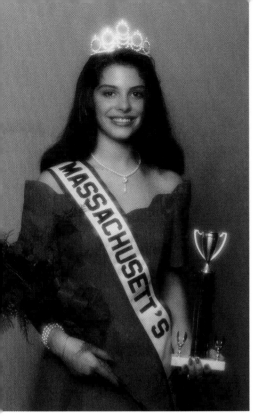

After I won my first pageant, Miss Massachusetts Perfect Teen. The dress was less than one hundred dollars from Filene's Basement.

career break: hosting *ET on MTV* and reporting for *Entertainment Tonight.*

My journey started with me working as a janitor and took me to NBC. I was raised in a non-English-speaking home by immigrant parents who had no formal education. I think I have above-average intelligence, but I'm no Rhodes Scholar. I was forty pounds heavier back then, too. I'm telling you all of this as proof that you don't have to be the smartest, richest, or prettiest to have success. You mainly have to work hard and have a positive attitude and passion—*no matter what the job.* The way I worked at Dunkin' is the way I work at NBC. Working like that will get you to NBC or wherever else you want to go.

EveryGirl Extra-Credit Tip: Not up for participating in a pageant? There are other organized gatherings that can be just as healthy, such as working on plays or engaging in musical competitions or sports. Again, you don't have to be a main player in any of these things if you don't have the confidence. You can be a supporting player and get the same positive results.

PAGEANTS WEREN'T SO BAD FOR MY BUSINESS, EITHER . . .

When you think of pageants, you think of psychotic mothers and their daughters fighting over a cheap tiara. The truth is that winning the crown is the least important part. Participating in pageants teaches you valuable skills that will serve you throughout life. By getting up onstage and addressing a crowd, you learn the art of public speaking. Before you get onstage, you have to solicit sponsors to raise money for entry fees. This doesn't teach you just about sales in the traditional sense—it teaches you how to sell yourself. Self-promotion is a big part of any career.

You also learn to get organized, set goals, and meet deadlines. You make new friends, too, and you learn about competition. You learn that not all the girls there are your friends.

Competition is a natural part of our lives. The earlier you embrace it and learn to cope with it, the better. I'm so thankful for my pageant experiences.

My job allows me to report on the red carpet and the sidelines, like here at the 2008 Super Bowl for the Patriots vs. the Giants.

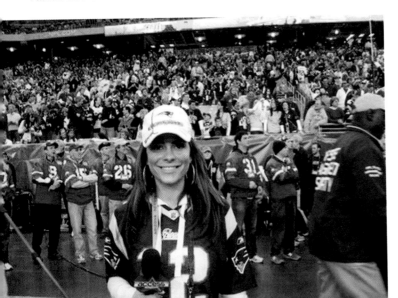

"Be confident. No matter what anyone else says or does, know what you stand for and what message you want the world to know; then say it over and over again. Make sure you are true to yourself at all times and believe in yourself. All these women are different and unique, but they all share an inner strength, and they know their inner compass and follow it. That's the secret to their success, and to yours!"

—Lucy Danziger, Self *editor in chief and coauthor of* The Nine Rooms of Happiness

Create a Life-and-Career Plan

Are you lost as to how to achieve your dream? Do you have so many things you like to do and accomplish that you don't know which way to turn? Join the club. Creating a career plan has helped guide me through it.

Remember the New Year plan (page 59) of writing out a game plan for your upcoming year? Well, the life-and-career plan is a plan for your upcoming life. You can do it along with your New Year plan, or you can do it right now. Take a blank piece of paper and create two columns on it. In the first column, write down what your ultimate career goal is. Where do you ideally want to end up? What do you want to be when you grow up? If it's a married mother of three, write it down. The plan will work for that, too. For example: *I want to be an entertainment reporter.* In the second column, list all the activities and projects you are currently participating in as well as the other goals and things you wish to do or achieve. Write down even little things that you invest your time and energy into on a daily, weekly, and monthly basis.

Start Making Cuts

Okay, now you should have your two columns. Carefully review and assess everything in column two. What you're looking for is which of these activities *most* support the realization of your ultimate goal.

Begin to order them numerically—number one helps you most to achieve your ultimate goal each number after that supports your ultimate goal less and less. Some will not support your ultimate goal; at all and even detract from it. You need to cross these off the list. But just because they're crossed off the list doesn't mean you won't be able to do them one day—just not now. When you're done with your list, you'll have a much better and clearer idea of what to prioritize in your life.

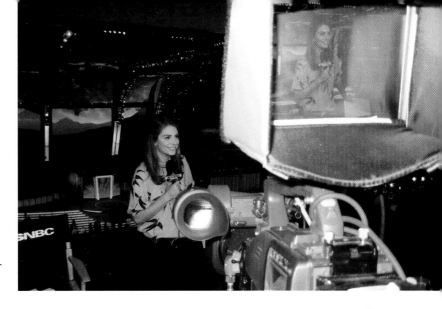

Here I am reporting for Access Hollywood *at the 2008 Democratic National Convention.*

Back to Your List

Hang the list up in a place where you can see it, and follow it for a year. Each New Year, review the plan and make amendments to it if need be. You may have new goals. The career chart is especially helpful for those who are good at, and like to do, a lot of things. Often, being good at many things splinters your time and focus and can inhibit you from reaching your ultimate goal. Having a list and seeing it will help.

EveryGirl Extra-Credit Tip: As part of your New Year plan, write out your life-and-career plan with the most trusted and knowledgeable member of your advisory committee. He or she can help you prioritize your goals.

GOD'S PLANS . . .

My friend Randal likes to repeat an old saying that if you want to make God laugh, tell Him that *you* have plans! In other words, things in life change. God continually puts new missions in our path, altering our plans. I find myself replotting my career plan during each New Year planning session.

The EveryMom at Work

I'm not a mom, but I come across a lot of working moms every day. It is truly a balancing act to keep it all together—but it is possible. Sure, there will be times when you have to give up stuff like field trips or when you might feel guilty about neglecting something. But learn not to be so hard on yourself! Remember your kids need quality time with a mother who remains positive and who takes care of herself. Because I'm not a mom, I asked some of my EveryGirl working moms how they do it all.

"We sit down together for dinner at least four nights a week. If I'm not there, I make sure they eat healthy and we talk about what happened at school that day."

—Lucy Danziger, Self *editor in chief and coauthor of* The Nine Rooms of Happiness

"I found a hobby that my kids and I would both like. When I saw how much my son loved birds, I realized bird-watching was something we could do together. We've taken great bird-watching excursions as a family to many places."

—Kate White, Cosmopolitan *editor in chief*

"When I come home from work, I really try to be with my kids. I help them with homework; we have family meals and play a game called Highlight-Lowlight, where we each tell our high point and low point of the day."

—Glynis Costin, InStyle *magazine West Coast bureau chief*

"Always find time to laugh, even in the most stressful circumstances. Lose your sense of humor and you've lost your day."

—Krista Smith, Vanity Fair *senior West Coast editor*

"Don't let work define you. Your family is the most important thing. I live for weekends. I don't make plans with friends. It's about my family and what my kids want to do. All my clients know I don't do activities at night. It's family time for me."

—Shelley Zalis, founder and CEO of OTX

EveryGirl Extra-Credit Tip: Having backup plans makes you more courageous, more confident, and more effective in your own work.

Diversify—Learn as Many Skills as You Can

Between the economy and the fast-paced world we live in, we are all being forced to wear more and more hats in our jobs today. Employers are expecting more, and we all have no choice but to deliver. The people who will survive are the ones who are multiskilled and are willing to apply those skills to their work.

Investment advisors always tell you to diversify, or have your money spread out in different areas, so if your real estate investment drops, you'll have your stock market investment to fall back on. You diversify in terms of your career for the same reason. Having extra skills and pursuing other work venues on the side are great ways to ensure you'll always have something to fall back on.

Starring alongside Sean Connery in From Russia with Love 007, *the Xbox video game.*

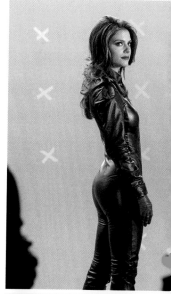

Backup Plans

The reason I learned how to do so many things—everything from makeup artistry to selling real estate—was because I'm a big proponent of backup plans. I've acted, produced, and directed films; done entertainment reporting and serious reporting; and am now writing books. Heck, if my entire career went sour, I could remodel and flip houses or, with my experience at Dunkin' Donuts, open a coffee shop. *Don't laugh!* I really want to one day. Having something to fall back on only makes me stronger and more confident and, therefore, more effective at whatever my current job is, too. My dad always says, "If you're a hard worker, you'll never be out of work."

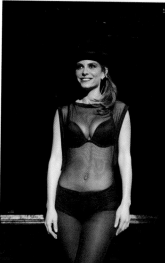

I've even gotten to perform on Broadway in a small role in Chicago.

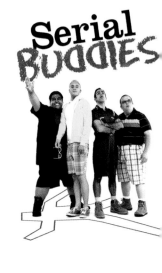

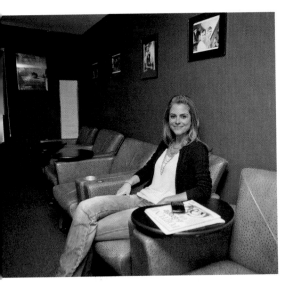

Getting ready to screen Serial Buddies, *which I produced and starred in. By the way, these are screening room chairs I got from my neighbor's trash.*

The Ecstasy of Defeat

Michael Jordan didn't make the varsity team in high school. The setback prepared him for the bumps ahead and fueled his drive to ascend to eventual greatness. I lost the Miss Massachusetts USA pageant. Months later, I moved to LA to report for Channel One and was at *Entertainment Tonight* soon after. Victory in the pageant would have consumed a year's worth of local commitments and prevented me from moving ahead in my career. Embrace your losses like you do your victories. If you do, you'll be rewarded by God, and your old friend the universe, and you'll discover they're just preparing you for a greater victory in the future.

And Don't Be Afraid to Work for Free

This is one that puts everyone in a tizzy, but I would *not* be where I am today had I not done this. I've worked for free, through junior high and into college, and I've always been rewarded for it. I worked for free for a year on my first movie, which got me to Channel One. When *One Tree Hill* offered me a part, the producers asked if I would do it for minimum pay, since they were overbudget that season. I laughed and told my agent that I'd pay them! I learned more about acting, and, today, people in other parts of the world know me just from seeing *One Tree Hill* reruns.

EveryGirl Extra-Credit Tip: A book that I found inspirational is *Letters to a Young Poet.* Pick it up—it may inspire your life-and-career path, too.

EveryGirl Extra-Credit Tip: Always send out thank-you cards to people you've interviewed with. It may be the thing to tip the scales and get you the job. Regardless, it leaves a nice impression.

Collect Contact Information

Be sure to get proper contact information from people you meet. Make a note on their business card where or how you met the person so you'll remember them when you see their information in the future. Ask them for their birthdays, too. You'd be surprised how many people are forgotten on their birthdays and how much they'll appreciate well wishes.

EveryGirl on the Job

A job is one thing, but a career is what we're really after. To have a career, you have to know how to work.

Be Positive at Work and Make It Fun

Remember what I did at Dunkin' Donuts, pretending to be Vanna and memorizing customers' orders? Most other successful self-made women were the same in their jobs. Rachael Ray is a great example. The girl wore nothing but a smile as she ran a tiny New York food store, enduring

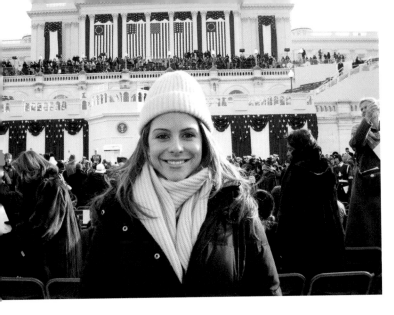

Keeping work fun is the key to getting ahead. If you like what you do, working hard for what you want is easier. Even in the bitter cold, I was all smiles while covering Obama's inauguration.

harsh conditions, such as cold early mornings and dangerous situations. These are the habits of successful people. Sure, negative, swindling jerks can succeed, too, but chances are greater they won't and you will *if* you're positive. No matter what the job was, and is to this day, I try to be positive and to make it fun. It's much better, and the work day goes much faster if I do.

Keep Busy

Remember that sense of urgency? You need it at work, too. You'll get more done in a day, have an easier time overall, and ascend for sure. If you don't have enough to do, check in with bosses to see if they need you to do anything. The key is to volunteer for more assignments instead of running away or hiding out when the work is done. Bosses appreciate this, and the day goes by faster, too.

EveryGirl Extra-Credit Tip: Watch biopics of successful self-made women like Rachael Ray, Bobbi Brown, and Diane Sawyer. Read their books, too. Study their habits and choices and emulate them. The example I used about Rachael was one I learned about through seeing a biopic on her.

"I don't pause too long on any single thing. If I can't solve something, I move on and come back later with fresh thoughts."

—*Lucy Danziger,* Self *editor in chief and coauthor of* The Nine Rooms of Happiness

Dinner Parties to Get Ahead in Your Career

Dinner parties can be affordable and fun ways to socialize. They're also the greatest means with which to network. I learned this from a big producer who today owns one of the nicest homes I've ever seen in LA. The producer started with nothing but had an innovative way to spark his career.

He used what small savings he had to throw one dinner party each week at his small apartment—hiring a cook who doubled as a server to do so. The cook-server gave the party a more formal presentation. For each dinner he would invite some people who were already successful, but mainly up-and-comers like him. It was an amazing, out-of-the-box, and super-creative way to meet new and diverse people and friends, as well as to network and further his,

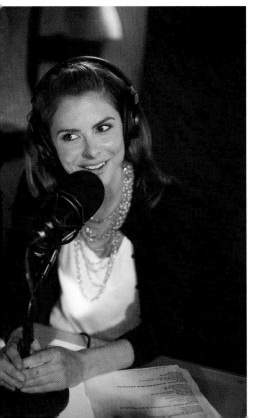

My team of experts—Rachel Zalis and Michael Russo and Tamara Ralph of Ralph & Russo—helps me choose the perfect dress for Emmy night. I'm so lucky to have reached a point in my career where my hard work is paying off in such exciting ways.

and everyone at the dinner's, careers. Host dinner parties of this kind. You don't need a server and can whip up something cost-effective yourself or with a coworker. And if you're invited to one of these parties, go!

Be Tech Smart

Did any of you see the performance of the former Illinois governor Rod Blagojevich on *Celebrity Apprentice*? He didn't even know how to turn on a computer, much less send a text message. You don't have to be a slave to every gadget that comes out either, but you need to keep in the know on current technology. There isn't a job I can think of where having this knowledge won't help.

Don't post inappropriate pictures of yourself or type anything you don't want to get out, either. Once it hits the Internet, it lasts forever. In the information age, future employers will surely check up on you and see them.

EveryGirl Extra-Credit Tip: Hit an Apple store to poke around to see what goodies they have and ask what they do. Also make an appointment at the Apple Genius Bar for help and check out their free classes.

Here I am hosting for AfterBuzz TV—a new media platform Keven created for TV and movie superfans worldwide.

Jealousy in the Workplace

We've all been there, having to deal with coworkers who for some reason or another just don't like us. We often think there's something wrong with us when, in reality, it might just be a case of jealousy. I asked EveryGirl expert Gina Marson to give us her advice for dealing with jealousy at work:

If a coworker is acting out of jealousy, either confront her directly by asking how you can work together more effectively or ask for advice from a trustworthy colleague. If your coworker appears to be jealous but is not acting out, ignore it. And don't engage in mind reading. It is not a good use of your time to begin wondering what she is thinking.

If it is you who is jealous, ask yourself what it is about your colleague specifically that is making you feel jealous. It could be that you are more competitive than you have admitted to yourself. You might need to accept your competitive nature. What you don't want to do is act out your jealousy against a colleague. Instead, focus on what *you* want to achieve.

Create Solutions, Not Problems

They say people are broken down into one of three parts at work: part of the problem, part of the landscape, or part of the solution. Be the one seeking to create solutions when problems arise. And never shoot down another person's solution or idea *unless* you have a better one to offer.

Stay Young

As I've stated, keeping a young heart is vital to all parts of life and growth, business included. Keeping up with technology, fashion, and grooming trends helps so much. That spirit of being open to growth and new things gives you energy and is just the spirit that keeps you employed. Older people who have young spirits are the ones who remain successful and relevant in their professions.

Invest in Yourself

Remember the outfit I bought for my Channel One interview? Remember the guy who hired a cook to throw dinner parties? Remember how I hired a publicist? In business, you have to spend some money to make money. Whether you need to buy a BlackBerry, a laptop, a printer, a desk, the right clothes, stationery, or even the right car, if it helps you to succeed and do better at your job, then don't be afraid to buy it. You're investing in your corporation. I've spent money on clothing, cars, exercise, office equipment, and electronic devices like PDAs, laptops, navigators, and even an iPad, for when I travel. All have helped make me more money in the end. When I've been cheap in this area, and I have, it's usually hurt me.

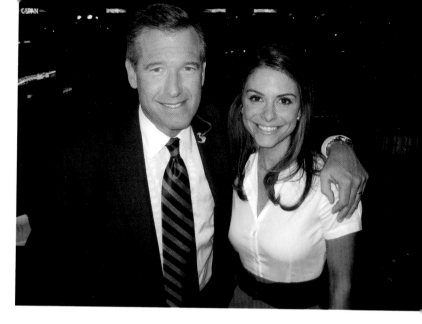

Brian Williams and me at the Democratic National Convention. Brian has been an amazing mentor and friend.

Seek Out Career Mentors

Their experience will expedite your success. To get the support of a mentor, you may need to give something of yourself to them—such as your time. There may be errands you can run and things you can do to help them. Having the right mentor, especially one who is powerful within your chosen career, is worth the efforts.

Stay on the Radar

It's always important to remain in touch with contacts and to remain on people's radars. Hitting them up on birthdays is great, but setting up a system where you can send out brief updates from time to time, or even annually, is better.

Use a running list to send holiday wishes to contacts, with updates on what you are doing. To be green and more cost-effective, send e-cards.

Man the F#@* Up!

One of my old agents cautioned me about asking for too much. He said a male A-list star can demand that his family, tutors, and nannies are all flown on private jets and put up in the finest hotels when shooting films. He can refuse to attend the premiere unless he's paid extra money. If a female A-list star demands the same, she's a bitch and a diva. These were very disheartening words.

So how do you get what you deserve or be tough when you need to without being labeled a bitch? You just have to be firm and state your case clearly and calmly without getting emotional. This is always a struggle for me. Friends say you get better with age. I am, and so will you.

A Quick Checklist of Maria's Career Dos and Don'ts

Quick Dos

- Be willing to work for free.
- Visualize the success you want to achieve.
- Always be looking to create solutions at work, not problems.
- Make the work that you do fun, no matter how miserable it seems.
- Wear a smile to work—and your best outfits, too (best *appropriate* outfits, that is).
- Try to be the first one in to work and the last one to leave.
- Focus on your own success, not your coworkers'.
- Learn the art of self-promotion.
- Embrace competition.
- Live your life as if you're going to run for president one day—this keeps skeletons from piling up in your closet.
- Take pride in, and have passion for, your work.
- Be resourceful, there's always a way.

Quick Don'ts

- Don't be a vampire.
- Don't put inappropriate comments or pictures on the World Wide Web. They are there *forever*.
- Don't shoot down ideas unless you have something better to put in their place.

And don't be afraid of losing popularity and the approval of others, either. I'm all for making the workplace a family environment, but take solace in knowing you have your parents, family, friends, and mainly yourself to give you all the love and support you need.

WORKING GIRL WEEKENDS

There's definitely a way to spend your weekends that's fun and healthy. The best weekends set you up for more success rather than detract from it.

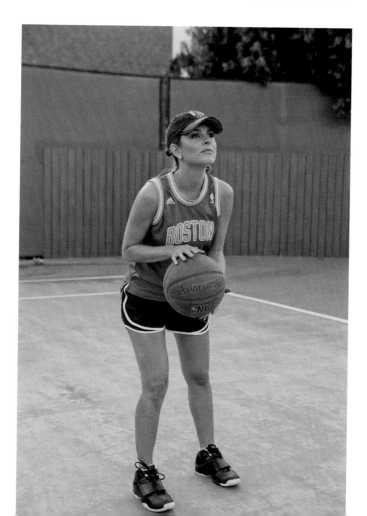

Think of your career as a game: Aim high and shoot for success.

EveryGirl Travels

The news has you traveling all over the place, and for me it's a few times a month. From packing, checking in, and going through security to making gate times, traveling is a stressful experience. It is imperative that I travel in a manner that's convenient, comfortable, and practical.

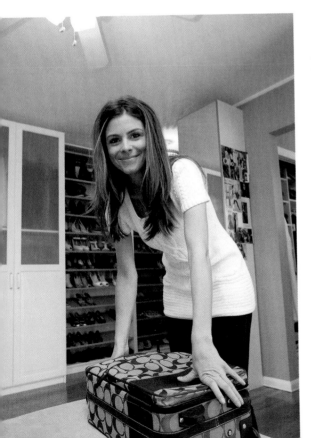

It's All in the Planning

Lazy people pack by just tossing a ton of clothes into bags at the last minute, figuring with quantity, they'll have what they need. But remember, lazy people work the hardest. Now they're lugging heavy bags—which may end up costing more to check—and when they arrive, they have more clothes to put away and sort through. They spend so much time picking out outfits and often don't have exactly what they need. The best way to pack is to do so the day before a trip, planning ahead what outfits you'll need and when you'll need to wear them and packing as little as necessary in the process.

Consider what you'll be doing each day and night on the trip. Lay out an outfit or outfits for

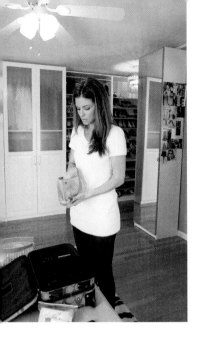

each day on your bed. Be sure to recycle different accessories—for instance, shoes and jeans, if jeans are appropriate—within each outfit.

"A good technique is packing according to color schemes. One trip might be my brown trip, and the next is the black. That means my basic clothes are all in one certain color. This way I can more easily mix and match pieces to create more outfits, while packing less."

—Shelley Zalis, founder and CEO of OTX

The EveryGirl Travel Checklist

Create a general standard checklist for packing. I have one on my Black-Berry and a printed one taped to the inside of my closet. This list has everything I'll need to travel, including toiletries, travel kits, passport, workout gear, headphones, computer, iPod, chargers, and cash. Create one that is tailored to your needs to ensure you don't forget things and to expedite packing. It's useful if a parent, partner, child, or assistant needs to pack for you, too. You can find my travel lists and more in the appendix.

Ready-Made Travel Kits

I have several ready-made travel kits that I'm able to just toss into my bag when I pack for trips. I use clear plastic makeup bags (they're great because you can run them through security), but I've used Ziploc sandwich bags from the supermarket, too. I have one each designated for toiletries, hair, and makeup.

Having the kits makes unpacking easier, as well. At the hotel, I simply take them out of the bag, and put them on the bathroom counter. At checkout time, I zip

My ready-to-go hair and makeup kits make it much easier on me to pack for a last-minute trip.

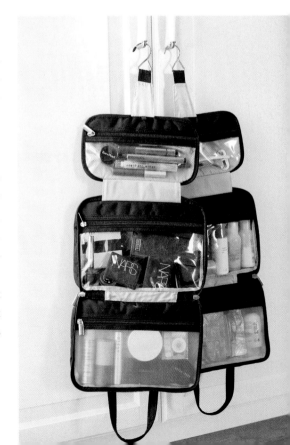

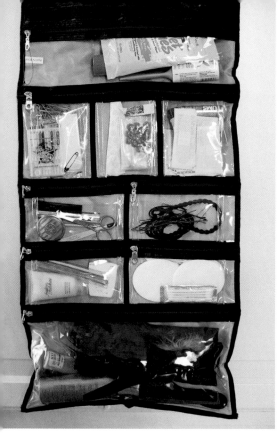

them back up, toss them in the bag, and then return them to my drawer at home, refilling as needed.

When purchasing your carry-on, look for a bag that not only meets airline requirements in size but also is constructed in a way that gives you the most interior bag space. More interior space means more room to pack clothes, which is crucial. Many bag interiors are cluttered with stuff like dividers and pockets that take up the room your clothes could use instead, so kick all the tires before buying.

I try to carry on my bags in lieu of checking in. With check-in, I lose time both in having to go to the ticket counter and, after deplaning, in waiting at the baggage carousel.

Your carry-on should be the proper size (check with airlines for size requirements) and on wheels so it's easy to transport. This bag will hold your clothing. A second bag should be either a backpack or large shoulder bag, for things you need during the flight, such as a computer, an iPod, headphones, magazines, a blanket, snacks, or medications.

EveryGirl Extra-Credit Tip: If you do check your luggage, in the event the airline loses it, be sure to pack important medications, your swimsuit, or anything else you can't go without in your carry-on.

A Maria Moment: "My-Pad"

For traveling, my iPad Wi-Fi + 3G is my lifesaver. On plane rides, I can watch videos, surf the Net, write down ideas, listen to music, read books, and access many helpful applications, too. It's much lighter than my laptop and takes up less space. I actually carry it in my purse at all times!

Downloaded and Ready

On the night before travel, download entertainment onto your iPod, iPad, or computer. You can download movies, podcasts, and TV series from iTunes. Some movies you can download for a rental period at rates as low

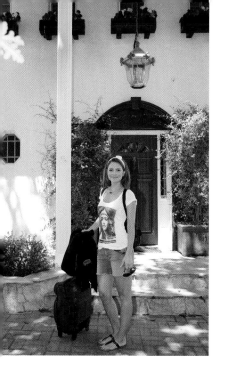

as $2.99. iTunes also has some amazing podcasts that you can download for free. Podcasts can be audio versions of your favorite news and talk shows, as well as informational broadcasts on any number of subjects (talk radio for the Web). Go to the podcast section at www.apple.com /itunes and type in a subject that interests you—reality shows, women's basketball, cooking, et cetera, and there is guaranteed to be a show that will be entertaining, informative, and perfect to listen to while flying. If you don't have an iPod, then save your money and get one! A few DVDs and your laptop, though bulkier, are great to set aside the night before travel as well. Be sure all phones, gadgets, and computers are charged.

A Maria Moment: Fashion on the Road

Less is more. I'm not afraid to wear jeans twice. One pair of jeans, comfy shoes, one pair of heels, and two or three tops, ranging from dressy to casual, go into my carry-on. Done! If I must pack more because it's a longer trip, then I'll ship my clothes to the location. Because I'm on TV, I need lots of different options! If you can't afford that luxury, then make sure it all fits in one bag.

"You want to be comfortable when flying, but I also believe in looking decent. You don't have to wear a suit, but don't wear sweatpants and a baggy old college sweatshirt, either. Have some lipstick and mints handy, too. And for the end of the flight, have some perfume to spritz on and a cover-up stick to eliminate your undereye bags before you head out to claim your other bags."

—Glynis Costin, InStyle *magazine West Coast bureau chief*

EveryGirl Extra-Credit Tip: Dermalogica sells skin-care kits with travel-size versions of their main products for $35. There's also a great website, 3floz.com, that sells only travel-size items.

EveryGirl Extra-Credit Tip: When packing, avoid accessories that take up a lot of room in your suitcase, such as big bracelets and purses. Small necklaces, earrings, and scarves are accessories that can be stored in plastic sandwich bags, rolled up, and inserted into shoes.

EveryGirl Extra-Credit Tip: If you're a TV junkie, go to iTunes and search for AfterBuzz TV to download some of our after shows. We break down episodes from your favorite TV series like *Mad Men* and *Dancing with the Stars*.

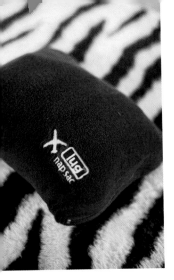

My travel pillow doubles as a blanket—just unzip it and voilà. I got this at the Container Store.

A Nightmare Maria Moment

A few years ago when I was flying home from Vegas, I had on this Express dress that was simple, summery, and comfortable. Perfect for airline travel, I thought. Well, it was until someone came up to me and said, "Excuse me, I don't know how to tell you this, but a guy just came up and took a photo underneath your skirt." I was horrified. How could I be so oblivious? Keven was with me, too, and he didn't notice it, either. This guy must have run up when neither of us were looking and snapped a shot and ran. The woman was able to point the guy out, and Keven couldn't help himself. He ran up to the guy, grabbed his camera, and deleted the pics. Airline officials were quick to do nothing. All I know is, I will never wear a dress to the airport again!

Must-Have Items for Little Emergencies

Always keep these with you on trips:

- Safety pins for rips and tears.
- A small sewing kit.
- ChapStick for your lips and flyaway hair.
- TOPSTICK to keep dresses or tops in place. You can also "hem" pants with it. The stuff is amazing for everything.
- Static Guard or a dryer sheet to avoid cling.
- A travel steamer. It's much cheaper than sending your clothes down to be pressed.
- Travel-size cosmetics, which are easy to transport. Buy little bottles from the Container Store and label them. There's nothing like washing your face with conditioner.
- Baby wipes. They can instantly fix makeup smudges and clean stains.
- Sanitizer gel to degerm everything.
- Mint chewing gum or travel-size toothbrush and toothpaste for bad breath after long flights.
- A multicompartment pill case filled with acetaminophen (for headaches), ibuprofen (body aches), and any other individual medications.
- A travel charger for your phone.
- A blankie/pashmina

Navigate the Airport with Ease

Getting through the airport is an art in and of itself. Here are some key things to know.

The E-ZPass

Many major airports have E-ZPasses now. E-ZPasses for frequent fliers allow you to bypass long lines and make airport travel easier. Check your airport's website for more info.

Online Check-in

If you have only a carry-on, check in online and print your boarding pass the night before. This prevents you from having to stand in long lines at the ticket counter. As soon as you get to the airport, you can head directly to security and the gates. Or use the self check-in kiosk if you do have bags. It's fast and easy.

Membership Has Its Privileges

Make sure to join your airline's frequent-flier club because this will often allow you to go through faster security lines or board before everyone else. If you travel a lot and can afford a membership to your preferred airline's lounge, it's worth it. For long layovers, or when you need to get work done, I find them very useful.

Going Through Security

Make sure to remember that you'll have to take off your shoes (don't wear complex boots), jewelry, belts, and the like, before you go through security. On travel days, try not to wear too many items that need to be taken off or clothes with a lot of buttons and studs. Studs may set off security alarms, which wastes time and is a huge pain. You don't want to be that person with fifty trays taking up all the space, either. As you approach security, grab your trays to be ready. Start unlacing shoes if they need it. Have your liquids (three ounces or fewer in those little bottles) in a clear plastic baggie. I'm always sure to place my liquids and my laptop on top of everything in my suitcase so that when I put my bag on the conveyor belt all I have to do is quickly unzip it and grab those items.

EveryGirl Extra-Credit Tip: Visit the website www.seatguru.com. You can type in the airline and flight number to get an exact description of your actual seat. They rate individual seats and give their exact size and dimensions. They also have all the specs on the plane itself, i.e., if it has Wi-Fi, TV, and meals.

EveryGirl Extra-Credit Tip: Tag your luggage with your phone number, not your home address. If your bag gets lost, someone can get in touch with you. And hold onto that baggage claim ticket, just in case.

EveryGirl Extra-Credit Tip: Stick to one airline for miles—mine is American but I also love Virgin America—and get credit cards that rack up miles, too.

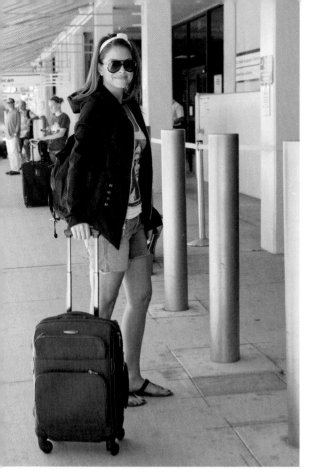

Going through security in this manner is simpler and far less stressful.

Eating at the Airport

It's easy to overeat at airports, but calories at airports count, too. The other day, I had greasy eggs and cheese on a sourdough bun when I landed. The stress and fatigue of travel can actually make your body crave sugary, fatty foods that will provide a quick, yet unhealthy, boost. Read a book or do some work on your computer instead of munching.

Boarding Flights

Before you board, you may want to take your laptop out of the suitcase if you intend on using it during flight. I have what I call an in-flight travel pouch. This is just a clear plastic, zippered travel bag made by Swissgear (a large Ziploc bag will work, too) that I fill with my iTouch, medications, gum, hand cream, or anything else I might need when in the air. I simply pull my travel pouch out from my bag and tuck it into the seat in front of me and I'm good for the duration of the flight.

A Maria Travel Moment

One flight, I passed out for the entire six hours. I woke up when we landed, wiping the drool off the side of my face. Yeah, I admit it, I drool sometimes! The guy next to me asked, "Are you famous or something?" I never know how to answer that question. I just said, "Why?" He said, "Well, everyone was coming up here to take pictures of you." I was like, "Oh great, I had to be drooling." No glam sleeping shots of me.

MARIA'S PLANE ETIQUETTE AND MUST-HAVES

- I always bring my own blanket. I use the plane blanket only if it's wrapped in plastic and clean.
- I have a pillow and blanket in one (see page 254) and a Tempur-Pedic SleepMask (sold on Amazon), a cushy mask to block the light when I want to snooze.
- Bring hand wipes and wipe down the armrests of your seat and the tray in front of you. I also have hand sanitizer that I can use with a napkin to wash my hands. It helps keep me from catching anything.
- I always drink hot water and lemon because I'm usually cold on the plane.
- Avoid dehydrating snacks, such as salted nuts and pretzels. Water-dense fruits and vegetables are excellent treats.
- Window seats are the best because I can lean up against the wall and sleep the entire flight. With an aisle seat, you risk being woken up when the passenger next to you needs to get to the bathroom.
- Bring headphones and your iPod on a plane to tune everything out or to enjoy your movies.

How to Avoid Conversations on the Plane

You can meet the most amazing and fascinating people when flying. I have. I've built lasting friendships with passengers and flight crews, too. But for the most part, flights are my time to catch up on work, to veg, and to recharge. I never check e-mails, since I want to close myself off from the world during this time. I sleep, read magazines, write, do research, and watch TV and movies, too. So what's my solution to avoid conversations? I keep my headphones on. It works for the most part, although I've had people tap me while I'm listening. I just try, as politely as possible, to get back to what I'm doing.

Here are my tips:

- Wear headphones.
- If you are first to arrive at your seat, when your seatmates come, don't make eye contact; this usually tells them you're not there to socialize.

- If they start a conversation, be polite and answer briefly but look right back down at your iPad, magazine, or book.
- If they get obnoxious then simply say, "I'm so sorry but I have a lot of work to do" or "I'm sorry but I really need to sleep" or "I really want to get back to this" (this being whatever it is you're doing).

Lost Baggage

When airlines lose your baggage, go right to the baggage lost-and-found office and place a report. After doing so, I usually spy around the baggage claim area, and inside the office as well, to see if my bag is, in fact, there. Too many times I've found it just sitting in those places, even though people behind the counter would tell me the bag was not at the airport and that they would call me if they found it.

Also, never pack valuables in your checked luggage. I once had all my jewelry stolen out of my bag because I didn't tip a really mean curbside guy. I knew who the guy was who stole my stuff and confronted him a week later when I was back at the airport. He denied it, of course, with a devilish twinkle in his eye. Inside, one of his colleagues came up and told me he saw his coworker steal my jewelry. I tried and tried with human resources to get my stuff back, but they couldn't have cared less. I learned my lesson though and hope you do as well.

And don't think because you put locks on your bags your stuff is safe. TSA officials can open anything.

Going to the Hotel or Airport . . . Ask for Women Drivers

Beware of drivers. If your company provides them, try and request the person you like or do as I do and request females. A few years back, I was heading home from the Grammys with a limo driver who had been inappropriate all night. Most drivers leave your bags on the front steps, and would never enter your home, but this driver followed me into my house, casing the area as he did. When he said, "So, you're all alone?" I knew this wasn't a good situation. What was this guy about to do? He worked for the top limo company in LA. This couldn't be happening—but it was. Knowing that a strong offense is a great defense in these situations, I yelled strongly, "Yeah, me and my big f-ing German shepherd!" All the while I'm thinking, *where the hell is Keven?* Just then, Keven came around the corner and said, "What's going on here?" The driver panicked and said, "Oh, I was just making sure she was okay," and then left quickly. If Keven hadn't been there, who knows what could have happened.

Ladies, please be careful. You are alone and vulnerable when picked up early in the morning or at night. Know who is driving you. If you don't, I highly suggest a female driver! I can't count how many bad experiences I've had with male drivers being inappropriate. In fairness, there have been some great male drivers, too. These are the ones I know and trust and who are recommended.

I don't always opt for limousines, either. Even though my work provides transportation for me, sometimes I opt to drive myself to the airport just to make it easier and to have more control. I often choose cabs over limos, too, during proper hours. In big cities, sometimes it's just easier to walk out of the airport and hail a cab.

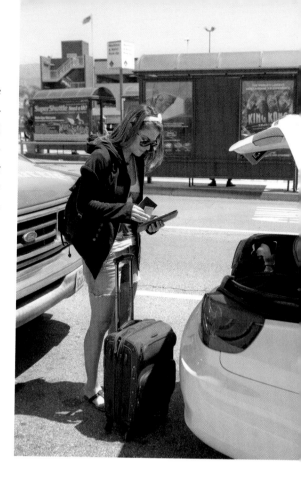

MARIA HOTEL TIPS

- Call ahead to the hotel and ask them what toiletries they provide. This will help you to lighten the load of things you need to pack.
- When staying at a hotel for more than two days, I'll visit the nearest store and stock up on bananas, water bottles, and pretzels, so when I'm starving I don't need to eat expensive hotel snacks. Hotel water can cost five times as much as what I pay at the convenience store.

EveryGirl Extra-Credit Tip: Shelley Zalis, a good friend of mine, asks the hotel in advance to clear out the minibar. (Ask the concierge.) This not only saves calories and money but also gives you a little fridge to store yogurt, cold water, and fruit, which you can buy cheaply at a supermarket in town.

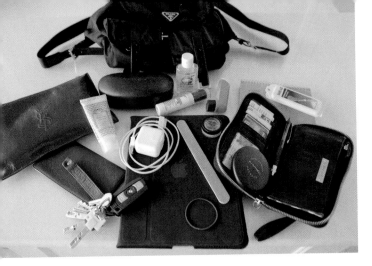

Travel essentials, like hand sanitizer, are very important!

Have a Travel Plan in Place at Home

Spur of the moment, you get a call from friends to hop on a plane and go away for the weekend. Who's going to water the plants, take in the mail, take out the trash, and feed the dog? The same goes for work-related travel. Have a plan in place for these occasions. There are services out there that do this very thing. The Pet Staff in Los Angeles, for example, will do all of the above *and* sleep over with the pets, feeding them and walking them for around seventy dollars a night. With your black book and all emergency numbers at hand, any house sitter or dog walker will be armed sufficiently so you can travel with peace of mind.

EveryGirl Extra-Credit Tip: Pack a small plastic bag to put dirty clothes in. When you unpack, just empty the dirty clothes into the hamper (or, if you really want extra credit, put them in the wash). It speeds up unpacking.

Unpack as Soon as You Get Home

Try doing this, even after four solid weeks of traveling, like I did recently. It's not fun, but it makes life so much easier when you do. Once I'm done unpacking and the suitcases are back in the closet, I feel such a relief and can fully enjoy being home.

The Vacation

When I hosted the Gracie Awards, an award show dedicated to powerful women in media, Suze Orman told all of us women to take more control over our money. She specifically mentioned not spending on frivolous vacations. Going on vacation is a blast, but I see too many girls blow thousands of dollars on them. This is money that could have served as down payments on condos or houses or could have just been better kept in the bank. For big vacations, wait for the right and responsible time in your life. When you live by the philosophy "work hard now so you can have an easy life later," you'll have enough money in the bank, and enough time, to splurge on a good vacation one day.

Other Great Travel Tips for the EveryGirl

- Bring ten to twenty one-dollar bills for tips.
- Organize all of your mileage accounts. Hotels like Starwood have great plans that allow you to earn free days. Keep all your numbers in your black book. Make sure you get credit for each plane ride and hotel stay. They really do add up—and quickly.
- Invest in a pocket translator if you're traveling overseas.
- Hide your passport or put it in a lockbox.
- Keep a medical-emergency card on you in case you get sick.
- Bring solid perfume sticks that easily fit into your purse. Security won't even hassle you about them, and it allows more room for other liquids in your baggie.
- Don't invest in high-end designer luggage. It will either get stolen or make your luggage a target for thieves. And keep an eye on your luggage in the airport. There are people who will walk by and try to take it "accidentally."
- Keep doubles of your essential toiletries (and other key items) with you in case things are lost. Buy a second phone charger.
- Take the hotel mini-toiletries for future trips. It's not stealing. They expect you to take them home.

On the positive side, vacations can be incredibly healthy, too. All sorts of studies indicate that going away on vacations can help women to be in better shape, live longer, work better, sleep better, and even have stronger marriages in the long run. The goal is to find ways to travel without compromising your finances and life.

The Friend-cation

Now that you are open to new friendships, you are bound to have friends all over the country and the world. Finding cheap flights and staying with them is the thriftiest vacation of all. The key to doing this successfully is to visit without being a bother to your friends.

Don't treat them like they're your concierges, having them schedule events, rides, and pickups for you. Renting a car at the airport is a worthwhile expense. This way you can come and go without bothering your host. Don't do anything to interrupt your friends' daily lives—remember,

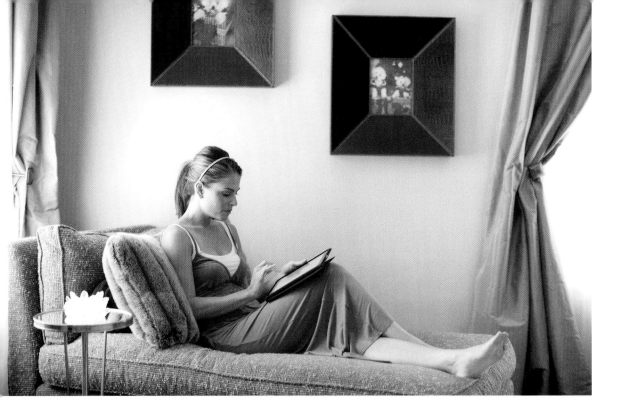

Sometimes vacationing at home is the best holiday of all.

you're the one on vacation, not them. Leave the apartment or house the same or better than it was when you arrived, and extend the invite back, expecting the same from them.

Flying out with a third friend (an equally considerate third friend) often helps the friend-cation—having a partner in crime to do stuff with takes more pressure off your host.

The Staycation

As I said earlier, many vacations serve to leave you only more exhausted and broke. The staycation, when you use your vacation time to stay at home and relax, is a healthy alternative to the rigors and expenses of travel.

Think out of the box. You can have people come to the house and give you massages or even cook for you, too. You can schedule something to do each day and night, e.g., visits to museums, concerts, amusement parks, sporting events, and shows. If you have children, you can do the same. I do my staycation around the holidays, since it's the only time I get off. I order food in, pull my couch out into a bed, gather the dogs, and just watch TV and movies all day and all night, dozing in and out of sleep as I do. It's amazing!

The Work-cation

This is my favorite kind of vacation and, between the economy and my lack of time, is pretty much the only kind I can afford to take. The work-cation is when you're sent away on work but get to have fun in the off-work hours or even stay an extra day or more to vacation. Your vacation is pretty much paid for by your company. If you have a job that involves travel, start seeing it as a work-cation. My friend Shelley Zalis, who is self-employed and therefore always dealing with work on her personal vacations, makes a point of only answering phone calls between 8 A.M. and 10 A.M. and at the end of the day. She keeps answering e-mails all day, though, to stay on top of things.

EveryGirl Extra-Credit Tip: You're going to indulge in great food and drinks on your trip. To keep the vacation pounds off, stay active. Engage in activities such as biking, walking, and other recreational and sporting activities.

The Weekend Vacation

I'm the kind of person who destresses with a quick weekend trip. That's enough time for me to enjoy myself and clear my head. It's cheaper, and I can do it more often than one big vacation.

Indicators That Your Travel Companion Is a Travelzilla

Be sure to travel with someone who enjoys doing the same things you do and has the right attitude. Too many vacations get ruined when, halfway through, you find yourself with a Travelzilla:

- They take forever to get ready. This will cut deeply into precious vacation time.
- They can't roll with the punches. Things go wrong on any trip. If they can't adapt, things will be much worse.
- They have no spontaneity. Trips are for escaping—which means being open to new things and adventures. A lack of spontaneity will kill this.
- They're negative and big-time complainers. The whole point of the trip is to have fun.
- They're cheapskates. Be smart and practical with your money, but being cheap is the antithesis of being on vacation.
- They're at a different life stage. They're single and want to meet guys and party till dawn; you want to relax and go to the spa on your vacation—or vice versa.

Avoid Needing a Vacation from a Vacation

I'm not one of those people who goes on vacation and comes back more tired than when I left. Vacation isn't about doing absolutely everything. It's far more important for me to rest than to scuba to the bottom of the ocean.

EveryGirl Extra-Credit Tip: Leave your BlackBerry in your hotel room when you're on vacation. Check it in the morning and at night.

If you like to party every single night on vacation, then you will leave needing a vacation from your vacation. Drinking will never help to rejuvenate you, but it is fun. Pad the end of your vacation period with one or two nondrinking days to allow time to recuperate. My perfect vacation is to leave on a Friday after work and be back the following Friday, so I still have Saturday and Sunday to recover. Most people come back late Sunday night and have to get up a few hours later for work. Or they have to stress over missing their flight, which would cause them to miss work. Don't end your relaxing vacation with all that unnecessary stress.

Partying Is More Fun When Done Less

The alcohol tastes better, the music sounds better, the company *is* better—better when you do it all less often. I have a weekend pool party for my birthday. I spend a lot of money, party like crazy, and have more fun than at weddings! I look forward to it every other year, and so do my friends. But if I did that every weekend, I know I wouldn't feel that way. I'd also be broke and in a hospital.

There are weekends I go to parties, but more than anything, weekends are there to realign and to recharge. I do that in a variety of ways that don't often involve drinking. I cook, bathe and walk my dogs, get a massage, work out, hike, read, hang with family and friends, play sports, do projects, shop, garden, hit matinee movies, and catch up on TV.

EveryGirl Extra-Credit Tip: Trade seasons of TV series with your friends and save money.

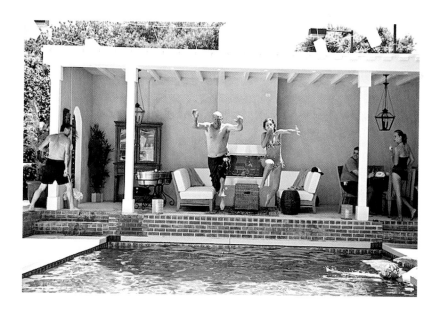

EveryGirl Gives Back

Life should be about giving. This means giving to your close friends and family but also giving back in charitable ways. It's a wonderful gesture that feels great. But gifts are always tough to buy for loved ones, friends, and relatives.

EveryGirl Plays Santa

EveryGirl Motto: Ask and you shall receive. Just say, "I'm looking for a gift for my boss. He's fifty and enjoys golf." I'm sure what you'll hear in return is "I have the perfect thing for you!"

I always do my holiday shopping in August. Why? It's usually the slowest month of the year for me, and the malls are less crowded than in December. I start with a spreadsheet of all the people I need to buy for. On the left, I list everyone who will be getting a gift. The next column is their age. And the next column is who they are to me: boss, friend, mom, dad, boyfriend, etc. The final column is what I end up buying for the person or what I plan to buy the person.

I do this because my list changes every year. People come and go in life. I also want to keep track of what I got people in the past so I don't get them the same thing and so I can know what level of gift they were sent or given. I keep this list on file, and the following year I update it.

I also like the spreadsheet because I can print it. It prevents me from forgetting anything and makes it easier to navigate through the mall. Some stores will have clerks available to help you identify the perfect gift for everyone on your list. Stores like Fred Segal in LA do this for me.

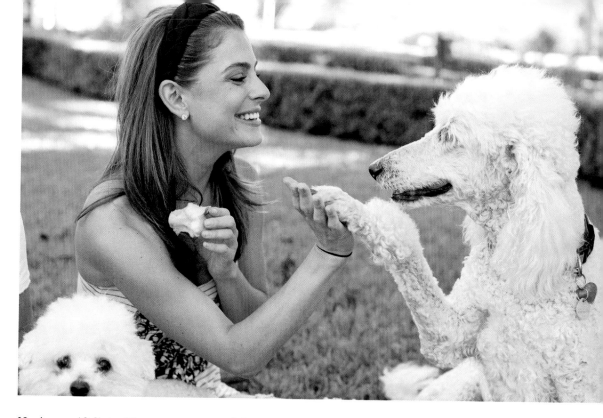

Having a gift list with names, ages, and descriptions is so helpful in this case. These assistants come at no added cost, nor do personal shoppers at large stores like Nordstrom. That aside, sales clerks in any store are likely to help you, either because they get a commission or because it's their job!

Tips For Buying Gifts

- Always tell the salesperson your price range. The last thing you want to do is overspend.
- Shop during the dead months, like early August, because the stores are empty.
- Remember that January is filled with great sales. Stock up on birthday gifts for the year.
- Have a small closet in your house (if possible) for those gifts, so you don't forget what you've bought.
- Don't be afraid to give another type of gift that costs much less. Invite someone for a home-cooked dinner.

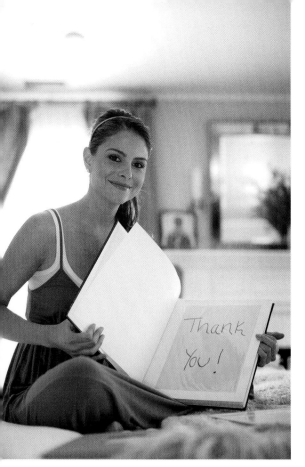

EveryGirl's a Scrooge

Don't be afraid to cancel Christmas or other gift-related holidays. I did it in 2009. I was so overwhelmed, so tired, and spread so thin financially that I just couldn't face it. I bought gifts only for those people who work closely for me. That was it! I chose to cook a big meal for friends and worked hard to make it a beautiful experience for everyone. Remember, days like Christmas aren't really supposed to be about gifts anyhow, unless you're a kid.

A Few of Maria's Favorite Gifts

A Thank-You Letter Book

Keven has everything, and the suggestions here don't apply to him anymore, because I've used them all up! So I get creative. Once, I had all his closest friends write him a letter describing what he means to them. Then I put all the letters together in a gor-

---

GIFTS THAT DON'T COST THAT MUCH

You might be scaling back on the gift-giving out of necessity. That doesn't mean you can't show love to your special people on the holidays or a birthday. Why don't you:

- Offer to walk their dog when they're on vacation?
- Offer to do some odd jobs for them, like helping get the yard ready for summer or driving them to the airport before a trip and picking them up?
- Offer to babysit five times in the next few months?
- Help them clean out their closet?
- Make a special picture book of memories or write them a heartfelt letter on what they mean to you?

geous scrapbook. Keven is a Tony Robbins selfless type who is always helping people but is rarely thanked for his efforts. So I had everyone he had helped write him a letter and, boy, did they get emotional. It was actually nice because sometimes people don't know how to thank someone and this provided them with a great opportunity to do it.

Needless to say, he cried when reading his scrapbook and said it was the best gift he ever received.

Now, What Do I Buy the Person Who Has Everything?

It's tough to buy for someone who has everything. In fact, I hear it all the time—"He [or she] has *everything*, so what could I possibly buy him [or her]?" Well, here are a few fail-safe items for anyone on your list:

- Slippers. UGG has some great ones for under fifty dollars. Brookstone sells form-fitting Tempur-Pedic Comfort-Step slippers that feel like heaven on your feet for under fifty dollars, too.
- A good, thick terry-cloth bathrobe, like the ones you get at high-end spas. I have so many and invite more. I love bathrobes. My mom got an amazingly soft one at Joblot!
- Throw blankets. My godchild and his family got me one for Christmas, and I love it.
- Snuggies are funny for someone who has it all and totally helpful for those who don't!
- Gift certificates. They're great for people who like to shop. Yes, they get a bad rap for not being personal enough, but I love them!
- Candles. They're amazing gifts because they come in all price ranges, and everyone loves a good candle. Voluspa is one of my favorite brands, but really any nice scent works. A candle is a really nice inexpensive gift that someone will use and appreciate but not necessarily buy for themselves!
- Costco always has nice wine and cheese baskets.
- Personalized anything. This can range from frames to stationery.
- A session with a personal trainer.
- Vintage candy in a gorgeous container. In LA, there's a store at Universal CityWalk that sells vintage-looking mailboxes. Fill them with popular old-fashioned candies. This is a great gift for guys and parents.
- A great coffee-table book
- Make your favorite cookies, then package them in a beautiful basket.

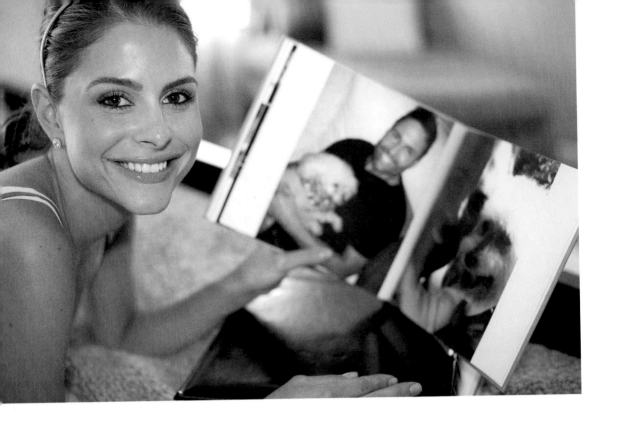

A Professionally Bound Picture Book

For Keven's birthday this past year, I gave him a photo album of our beloved poodle, Noelle, who had died earlier that year. Losing her was like losing a child. Knowing most guys don't make photo albums, I compiled all the photos I had of his journey with Noelle and went to the Kodak Gallery online. Through the site, you can submit your photos, along with any captions you'd like to write. For as little as twenty dollars, they create a coffee-table album book for you. The Noelle memory book was another tearjerker and remains at his bedside.

Memorabilia

If you know someone who collects memorabilia (no hoarders please!), that's always a thoughtful route, too. Sometimes you can find a gem for cheap, and it shows you were actually listening when they said, for example, "I'm a big fan of the show *24*." You can search online for memorabilia sales. It's fun searching for the perfect thing, and you'll learn a little about what your friend likes so much!

Handmade Is Best Made

By the way, anything handmade rocks. My assistant this year made me chocolate chip cookies and packaged them in a super-cute little Christmas container. "Genius," I thought. It was inexpensive and showed me that she cared enough to make me something—and the cookies were delicious.

It's All in the Packaging

Packaging really makes a difference, too! Homemade cards are always fun. A friend took an old shoebox and designed it to double as a gift box and a card. So be creative. It's fun and cheap! And sometimes it's green, too!

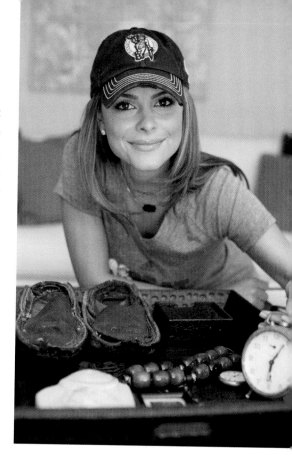

I love keeping little artifacts from my family. These are my dad's shoes, made from tires, that he wore in Greece.

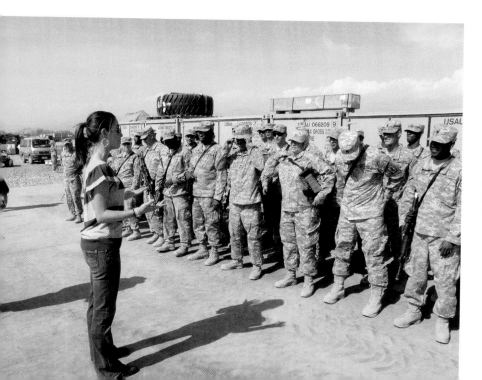

Here I am on base in Afghanistan, thanking the troops for their sacrifice and service.

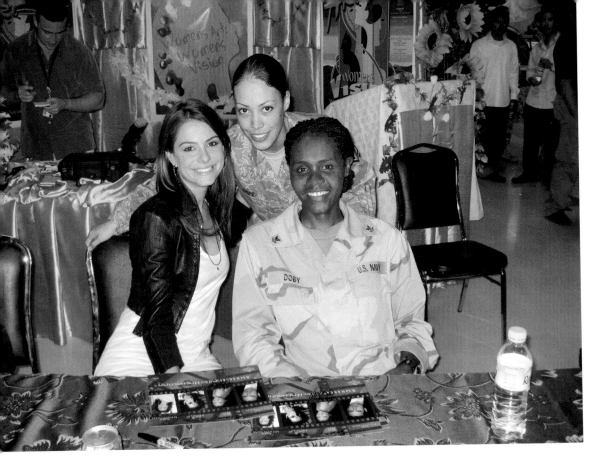

In March 2008, I visited the troops in Afghanistan.

A MARIA MOMENT

Give a gift that gives back. For Christmas 2008, I issued a challenge on behalf of my charity, Take Action Hollywood. I asked people to buy only gifts that give back, gifts from companies that donate proceeds from sales to charity.

This is what I wrote on the website, asking others to give:

"As we approach the next holiday season, I am asking you to participate in my Take Action Hollywood! Holiday Challenge when shopping for gifts this season. The challenge is to purchase gifts and products from select companies that specifically designate portions of the sale/proceeds of the gifts to charities and charitable causes. It's the way I'm shopping this year, and I hope you'll follow suit."

Maria's Charities

Here's a list of current causes close to my heart:

- Diabetes—I work with EIF, the Entertainment Industry Foundation. As the Diabetes Aware Ambassador, I make countless trips to Capitol Hill on behalf of EIF to educate and rally support for diabetes.
- Animal charities—I try to promote pet adoption and try to help prevent cruelty to animals through various organizations I donate my time to.
- Children—I work with the children's hospitals in Boston and Los Angeles to brighten kids' days and get them much-needed money and donations, as well as sponsor and host my annual day of beauty event where I bring the top makeup and hairstylists in to make over the kids.
- The troops—I love our troops and flew to Afghanistan to visit with them. It was a moving experience and I am planning my next trip as we speak.

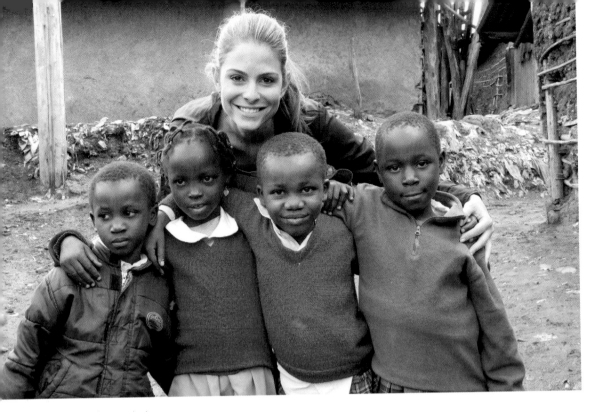

Here I am in Africa with the girls of the Kibera School for Girls.

EveryGirl Gives Back

Since I was thirteen, I've been trying my best to give back. For my church, the Dormition of the Virgin Mary Greek Orthodox Church, I was president of the youth group, which was called GOYA, and sang in the church choir. While president of GOYA, we caroled at local nursing homes and held numerous fund-raisers, too. Through the pageants I was involved in, I worked with the Special Olympics, among other causes. I also volunteered at the Malden Hospital, in a city next to my hometown. At the hospital I would visit with patients and read to them. I loved it and in the process I met some wise elders who gave me great advice.

Giving really does go both ways. Volunteer work helps puts life in perspective and makes you appreciate what you have. It blesses you with good karma and is also a free training ground, helping you to attain useful skills that will set you up for success. My volunteer work taught me how to produce and organize events and how to motivate people behind a cause. These are skills I use in producing TV programs and movies, as well as in so many other areas of my life. I also made great friends and contacts and certainly received my healthy share of good karma, too. There is no way I would be successful had I not given back. I still do my best to give back today and still get the same amazing results each time I do. One of my goals is to do more when I retire.

By the way, anyone can do volunteer work. You don't need to be educated, rich, or famous. Old or young, rich or poor, anyone can volunteer and give back and receive blessings in return.

My friend Randal says the only reason we're really here on earth is to help one another, and I believe that's the right way to look at life. It's no coincidence that this is the last paragraph of the book. Last impressions are often what we remember. If all you're left with is the notion that your purpose here is to help people—and you live up to that purpose—then you've learned enough to be successful.

OTHER WAYS TO GIVE BACK

- Volunteer to work in an old-age home or a children's hospital. You can talk to families and even reap the advice of wonderful seniors. I learn so much from elders, and this helps me to refrain from making mistakes.
- From your friends, collect clothing and toys to donate to a local women's shelter.
- Stage events that raise money to give to worthy charities in your area and around the world.
- Participate in walks for cancer and other diseases. They're a great way to earn money for wonderful causes, plus get exercise.
- Work to clean up the natural areas of your town. Many women have banded together in urban areas to clean up parks, which are now gorgeous for everyone.

Acknowledgments

On my first call with Lisa Sharkey and Amy Bendell of HarperCollins, I was advised to hire a ghost writer. A what?? I never knew that people didn't write their own books. I interviewed a few writers and quickly realized this was definitely not going to work. The book is far too personal. Plus, I really, truly wanted to share *everything* I've learned in my journey with you guys. Lisa and Amy grew nervous and rightfully so. Someone with as many jobs as me surely wouldn't be able to meet deadlines and surely would need help. I approached the best writer I knew. Someone who knew me better than anyone. Someone who has been on the journey with me. Someone who has taught me many of the lessons I share in this book. That someone is Keven Undergaro, my partner in crime for the last twelve years. We started out together making movies out of a basement in Boston. Since then, Keven has been my advisor, mentor, and partner the entire way. Funny thing is, I call him my memory bank because he's the one who remembers my red carpet moments better than I do. However, though he has written plenty of TV and film scripts, he'd never written a book. With our minds in our usual states of "possibility" we decided to team up and write it together. We called Lisa and Amy, pled for patience and guidance, and off we went. We fought tons. But in the end, I think we did a good job. Aided, of course, by many people along the way and for them I'm truly grateful.

Thank you, Lisa Sharkey, Amy Bendell, Frank Weimann, all of my EveryGirl experts, Kathleen Indigaro, Sophia Carafotes, Mary Carafotes, Margo Popken, Startraksphoto.com, Cindy Pearlman, Corey Sheehan,

Meredith Ahern, Melodie Moore, Valerie Fatehi, Jami Kandel, Rob Silverstein and everyone at my NBC family, Alan Berger and CAA, Special Artists, and everyone at HarperCollins who worked so hard on this book.

Cate Hemingway, your positive energy, hard work ethic, and constant support has been a blessing that has improved my life tremendously. Thank you!

One major shout out to Elise Donoghue. This book was never meant to be in color. Your sensational photos made this book what it is. Now women don't have to just read how I do things, they can see it. Thank you for your patience, time, and extraordinary talents. Most of all, thank you for your friendship.

This book also wouldn't be possible without all of the experiences and lessons leading up to my journey to Hollywood. Growing up in Medford was wicked awesome. I thank the city, and my schools and teachers, for helping to groom me into who I am today. Teachers are the foundation for everything we are and become, and they unfortunately are not revered enough, not to mention paid enough, for what they provide. Thank you for teaching me how to speak English, Ms. Brenner!

Thank you to my church, the Dormition of the Virgin Mary Greek Orthodox Church. I loved every second I spent there and thank everyone who ever advised me. What a great community to have grown up in and as you'll read in the book, my lessons in producing and multitasking started there.

Thank you to Emerson College for my great education in media and film. I can't speak more highly of a school that does more to keep their students on the cutting edge and provide them with the tools to be the best.

Thank you to the Miss Massachusetts Teen/USA system. Laurie Clemente, I will forever cherish our times together. Thank you for wrapping your arms around me and teaching me lessons I still utilize today.

Thank you to my cousin Anthony Menounos. Without you, my parents would have never let me compete in the pageants, nor would they have allowed me to live at college; two experiences that helped me get to where I am today. Your support in those years meant everything to me and still does.

Thank you to my parents. Dad, I know I sometimes laugh at your stories about not having shoes and walking six hours in the snow just to get to school, but I appreciate it. Thank you for drilling lessons into my brain and for encouraging me, "Maria, you can do anything you put your mind to." Well, I believed you, Dad, and here we are. Mom, your tireless support taking me to every fashion show, every pageant, every modeling gig all the while working in the school cafeteria, maintaining the house, and keeping Dad alive through all his low blood sugar attacks. I will forever be grateful for your sacrifices to help me get here. The things you've been subjected to, witnessed, and experienced are so difficult to speak about and yet you always have a smile and are always positive. You're an inspiration and a great model of strength. You guys both killed yourselves to provide me with a better life, thank you and I love you.

And to Keven, without you there is no journey. Tears well in my eyes when I think of how much you've helped me. There really is no way to explain what you've done for me and my family—that's another book in itself. I would never be where I am today without you. You helped me succeed in a brutal business. You told me it was possible to act and report for the news. I was scared, but you knew better. You've set aside your journey and your work to help me achieve my dreams. You selflessly have taken a backseat for twelve years. Thank you for believing in me and investing in me. I've never met anyone so giving and so kindhearted and yet at the same time so misunderstood. I'm in the presence of greatness every day and I cannot wait for your turn in the sun. I cannot wait for everyone to see the genius I see and experience every day. Your turn is coming.

Thank you for helping me write a great book. Together, we became authors. Minds in possibility always! I'll never forget when Joan Rivers said she wished she had a champion in her corner. Thank you for being mine. I love you.

Thank you, Alyssa, for being my best friend since seventh grade and for always being there; Joe, for being a great big brother; and Nancy Ranzo, for opening your home to me at a time when I needed it most.

For my LA journey, thank you, Rachel Zalis, for being the big sister I never had but always wished for. Thank you to Kevin Yorn, Gary Mantoosh, and Alix Gucovsky, you all have been there with me since the beginning. I might not have gotten this far without you.

And thank you to the EveryGirls out there who have followed my career and supported me along the way.

EveryGirl Experts

Many thanks to all the EveryGirl experts who helped fill this book with useful information and tips. I have learned so much from these amazing women, and I am glad I could share their wisdom with you.

Jake Bailey, celebrity makeup artist

Bret Boreman, celebrity makeup artist

Nicole Bryl, makeup artist to the stars, Make-up New York

Glynis Costin, *InStyle* magazine West Coast bureau chief

Tommy Cyr, celebrity hairstylist

Lucy Danziger, *Self* editor in chief and coauthor of *The Nine Rooms of Happiness*

Olivier Geymann, stylist at Serge Normant at John Frieda Salon in Los Angeles

Valerie Hunt, celebrity makeup artist

AJ Jolivette, CTO/president, Soho Network Services, Inc. IT You Can Trust

Dr. Raj Kanodia, a well-respected international plastic surgeon from Beverly Hills

Annet King, director of global education, the International Dermal Institute and Dermalogica

Stacy London, cohost of TLC's *What Not To Wear* and cofounder of Style For Hire

Dr. Gia Marson, psychologist

Melanie Mezzacappa, celebrity hairstylist

Andrea Orbeck, fitness specialist

Mariolga Pantazopoulos, celebrity makeup artist and hairstylist

Dr. Gail Saltz, psychiatrist and psychoanalyst

Krista Smith, *Vanity Fair* senior West Coast editor

Anastasia Soare, CEO of Anastasia Beverly Hills

Kate Somerville, founder of Kate Somerville

Patti Song, hair color expert, represented by Cloutier Remix

Kate White, *Cosmopolitan* editor in chief

Kyle White, celebrity colorist of the Oscar Blandi Salon in New York

Yogi Cameron, author of *The Guru in You*

Rachel Zalis, fashion expert

Shelley Zalis, founder and CEO of OTX

Appendix

Your Little Black Book

To get you started on your way to creating your own black book, I have included the lists I use and find helpful.

My black book is divided into the following sections. Each section has its own tab in my binder. Feel free to use this as a guide and add sections that work for you and your life.

Birthdays (and other important dates)

January	
February	
March	
April	
May	
June	
July	
August	

September	
October	
November	
December	

Work Info

Company Name:
Address:
Phone:
Fax:
Federal Tax I.D. Number:

Accountant:	
Airlines:	
Airport Greeter:	
Artwork Shipping:	
Attorney:	
Bank:	
Blackberry:	
Car Service:	
Cell Phone:	

Computers:	
Courier:	
Credit Cards:	
Florist:	
Framing:	
Gift Baskets:	
Health Insurance:	
Insurance:	
Messenger:	
Photo:	
Portfolio Supplies:	
Printer Repair:	
Printer Supplies:	
Stationery:	
Telephone:	
Travel Agent:	
Video Reel:	
Website:	

House

Vendors	
Alarm:	
Realtor:	
Attorney:	
Camera (Surveillance):	
Cleaning Service:	
Contractor:	
Electricity:	
Exterminator:	
Plumber:	
Insurance:	
Landscapers:	
Management:	
Mortgage:	
Pool Man:	
Snow Removal:	

Housekeeper:	
City Hall:	
Car Company:	

Key passwords

Vendors	Passwords
BlackBerry:	
AT&T:	
Kodak Gallery:	
Twitter:	
Labites:	
FedEx:	
New York Times Web:	

Imdb:	
Gogo Inflight:	
Directv:	
Luggage Locks:	
Outdoor Lockbox:	
Bank Accounts:	

Emergency Contacts:

Friends/Family

Friends	Phone #

Family	

Travel Info

Car Company:	
Boston:	
Los Angeles:	
Airlines:	
To Boston:	
To New York and Elsewhere Domestically:	
Hotel:	
New York:	
Boston:	
Airline Mileage Accounts: Maria:	
American Airlines:	
United Airlines:	
Virgin America:	
Delta:	
US Airways:	
Continental:	

Passport Number	
Driver's License Number	

Personal Information

Legal Information	
Legal Name:	
Date of Birth:	
Social Security:	
Mother's Maiden Name:	
Passport Number:	
Driver's License Number:	
Contact Information	
General:	
LA House:	
Connecticut House:	
Family Information	
Parents:	

Sibilings:	
Other	
Bank Accounts:	
Credit Cards:	
Safety Deposit Box:	
Medical Information:	
Health Insurance:	
Doctors	
Primary Care:	
Gynecologist:	
Dermatologist:	
Therapist:	
New York Doctor:	
Dentist:	
Chiropractor:	
Pulmonary Specialist:	
Heart Specialist:	
Colonoscopy:	

Podiatrist:	
Diabetes Specialist:	
Prescriptions	**Prescription Number**
Pharmacy:	
Miscellaneous	
Laser Hair Removal:	
Trust Lawyer:	

Contact List

Pool Man:	
Computer:	
Electrician:	
Gardener:	
Interior Design:	
Party Planner:	
Pharmacy:	
Housekeeper:	
Security:	
Handyman:	
Spa Repair:	
Pest/Rodent Removal:	
Cable:	
Glass/Windows:	
PO Box:	
Junk Removal:	
Fountain Repair:	

Treadmill Repair:	
Home Entertainment/TV/Music Guy:	
Realtor:	
Home Warranty Info:	
Internet:	
Plumber:	
Corvair Repairer:	
Mechanic:	
Gate Repair:	
Garage Doors:	
Gate Motor Company:	
AC Technicians—Annual Service:	
Pool Contractor:	
Phone:	
Christmas Lights Installation:	
Hardwood Floors (Burbank St.):	

Travel Checklist

Toiletries

- [ ] Toothbrush
- [ ] Travel-size toothpaste
- [ ] Dental floss
- [ ] Travel-size mouthwash
- [ ] Travel-size deodorant
- [ ] Razor
- [ ] Travel-size shaving cream
- [ ] Travel-size shampoo
- [ ] Travel-size conditioner
- [ ] Travel-size soap
- [ ] Botanical cream for dry hair
- [ ] Travel-size thickening spray for hair
- [ ] Travel-size hairspray
- [ ] Travel-size makeup remover
- [ ] Travel-size SPF for face
- [ ] Travel-size face wash
- [ ] Travel-size face toner
- [ ] Travel-size face moisturizer
- [ ] Travel-size cleanser
- [ ] Travel-size facial scrub
- [ ] Travel-size facial mask
- [ ] Eye treatment/cream
- [ ] Travel-size saline solution
- [ ] Contacts case
- [ ] Makeup remover towelettes
- [ ] Roll-on perfume
- [ ] Travel-size sunscreen
- [ ] Feminine-hygiene products
- [ ] Tampons

Miscellaneous Travel Toiletries

- [ ] Antibacterial wipes
- [ ] Tissues
- [ ] Travel mirror
- [ ] Static Guard
- [ ] Lint roller
- [ ] Safety pins
- [ ] Travel-size sewing kit
- [ ] Foot cushions
- [ ] Double-sided stick tape
- [ ] First-aid kit
- [ ] Band-Aids
- [ ] Travel-size lotion
- [ ] Cotton pads and cotton balls
- [ ] Q-tips
- [ ] Assortment of makeup brushes

Medications

- [ ] Advil
- [ ] Vitamins
- [ ] Birth control
- [ ] Pain reliever
- [ ] Denavir
- [ ] Benadryl
- [ ] Tums
- [ ] Inhaler
- [ ] Tweezers
- [ ] Scissors

Hair products

- [ ] Hair brush
- [ ] Comb
- [ ] Hair dryer
- [ ] Curling/flat iron
- [ ] Bobby pins

- ☐ Elastic hair ties
- ☐ Headbands

Nail Products

- ☐ Nail file
- ☐ Nail clippers
- ☐ Nail polish remover

Makeup

Skin/Face

- ☐ Translucent powder
- ☐ Foundation stick
- ☐ Bronzer
- ☐ Color corrector kit
- ☐ Foundation
- ☐ Portable powder stick with SPF
- ☐ Pot rouge for lips and cheeks
- ☐ Leg makeup/self-tanner

Eyes

- ☐ Assorted eye shadows in various colors
- ☐ Gel eyeliner
- ☐ Liquid eye color
- ☐ Eye powder

- ☐ Mascara
- ☐ Water-resistant eye shadow
- ☐ Eye pencil
- ☐ Eye concealer
- ☐ Brow powder
- ☐ Clear eyebrow gel

Lips

- ☐ Assorted lip glosses in various colors and shines
- ☐ Lip balm
- ☐ Lip pencil

Travel Necessities and Accessories

Basics

- ☐ Travel aids
- ☐ Pleasure reading
- ☐ Chewing gum
- ☐ Snacks
- ☐ Bottled water
- ☐ Earplugs
- ☐ Sleeping mask
- ☐ Travel pillow
- ☐ Motion-sickness remedy

- ☐ Sleeping pills
- ☐ Anxiety medicine

Funds

- ☐ Wallet
- ☐ Cash
- ☐ Credit cards
- ☐ ATM card
- ☐ Traveler's checks

Travel Info

- ☐ Passport and visas
- ☐ Driver's license
- ☐ Itinerary
- ☐ Maps and directions
- ☐ Travel tickets
- ☐ Travel confirmations
- ☐ Travel membership cards
- ☐ Travel guides

Documents

- ☐ Copies of travel documents
- ☐ Copies of credit cards
- ☐ Copies of passports
- ☐ Credit card contact info
- ☐ Emergency contact info

- ☐ Medical insurance card
- ☐ Medical history
- ☐ Prescriptions
- ☐ Travel insurance
- ☐ Car insurance card

Bags

- ☐ Backpack/day bag
- ☐ Purses
- ☐ Collapsible tote
- ☐ Money belt
- ☐ Shoulder straps
- ☐ Plastic bags

Laundry

- ☐ Laundry bag
- ☐ Laundry kit
- ☐ Stain remover
- ☐ Travel iron

Miscellaneous

- ☐ Umbrella
- ☐ House keys
- ☐ Travel locks and keys
- ☐ Luggage tags
- ☐ Hospitality gifts
- ☐ Journal
- ☐ Sports gear

Contacts

- ☐ Address book
- ☐ Important numbers
- ☐ Datebook
- ☐ Business cards
- ☐ Calling card

Technology

- ☐ Cell phone and charger
- ☐ PDA and charger
- ☐ Laptop and charger
- ☐ Camera and charger
- ☐ Film
- ☐ Music and player
- ☐ Headphones
- ☐ Voltage adapters
- ☐ Batteries
- ☐ Flashlight
- ☐ Binoculars
- ☐ Alarm clock

Work

- ☐ Work documents
- ☐ Work reading
- ☐ Office supplies
- ☐ Notebook

Clothes

Basics

- ☐ Underwear
- ☐ Socks
- ☐ Undershirts
- ☐ Bras
- ☐ Pantyhose
- ☐ Sleepwear
- ☐ Robe

Dressy

- ☐ Dress shirt
- ☐ Sweaters
- ☐ Blazers
- ☐ Slacks
- ☐ Skirts
- ☐ Dresses
- ☐ Suits

Outerwear

- ☐ Jackets
- ☐ Coats
- ☐ Raincoats
- ☐ Hats
- ☐ Gloves
- ☐ Scarves

Casual

- ☐ T-shirts
- ☐ Tank tops
- ☐ Sweatshirts
- ☐ Jeans
- ☐ Shorts
- ☐ Exercise clothes
- ☐ Swimsuits

Footwear

- ☐ Athletic shoes
- ☐ Leisure shoes
- ☐ Dress shoes
- ☐ Sandals/flip-flops
- ☐ Slippers

Accessories

- ☐ Belts
- ☐ Ties
- ☐ Wristwatches
- ☐ Jewelry
- ☐ Glasses
- ☐ Sunglasses
- ☐ Reading glasses
- ☐ Glasses cases

Essential Supplies for the EveryGirl's Office

Ink Cartridges

- ☐ Color 97
- ☐ Black and white 96
- ☐ Reams of paper
- ☐ Manila folders
- ☐ Hanging file folders
- ☐ Paper clips
- ☐ Pens
- ☐ Post-its
- ☐ Notebooks
- ☐ Tape

Stack and Attack Lists

Before you go shopping, make a list of the things you need. Here's an example to get you started:

Food

- ☐ Turkey deli meat 1lb
- ☐ Roast beef deli meat 1lb
- ☐ White cheddar 1lb
- ☐ Mustard
- ☐ Bread
- ☐ Greek yogurt
- ☐ Skim milk
- ☐ Soy milk
- ☐ Peanut butter
- ☐ Cut celery/carrot sticks
- ☐ Romaine salad bag mix
- ☐ Hummus
- ☐ Cereal
- ☐ Granola
- ☐ Blueberries
- ☐ Blackberries
- ☐ Cantaloupe

- ☐ Watermelon
- ☐ Mixed nuts and peanuts
- ☐ Sodas

Cabinet and Medical

- ☐ Oval cotton pads
- ☐ Makeup remover wipes (Neutrogena)
- ☐ Kleenex/cube boxes
- ☐ Mini tissue packs
- ☐ Calcium with Vitamin D
- ☐ Vicks Vapor Rub
- ☐ Mouthwash
- ☐ Theraflu
- ☐ Band-Aids
- ☐ Gauze pads

- ☐ Sudafed nasal congestion remedy
- ☐ Rubbing alcohol
- ☐ Motrin
- ☐ Advil
- ☐ Emergen-C
- ☐ Zicam
- ☐ Tylenol PM
- ☐ Coldcalm
- ☐ Cold-Eeze
- ☐ Tylenol cough and sore throat
- ☐ Tums
- ☐ Tylenol extra strength
- ☐ Wet Ones

- ☐ Mucinex
- ☐ Iron
- ☐ Claritin
- ☐ Benadryl
- ☐ Zantac
- ☐ Baby powder

Dog and Cat Supplies

- ☐ Cat food
- ☐ Dog food
- ☐ Dog snacks
- ☐ Cranberry Relief
- ☐ Pee Pads

Food Charts

When trying to lose weight, keeping track of what you eat is important. Here are some examples of my food charts from back in the day. This is exactly what I ate.

Date Friday 9/17/99	Protein	Carbs	Fats	Calories
Breakfast				
grapefruit				
3 eggwhites mush/onion		15	0	75
2 graham	2	23	1.5	110
Mid Morning				
Lunch				
salad w/ chicken	31	0	4	165
1 pita bread				
dressing				
Mid afternoon				
apple	0	21	0	81
2 cups tea	0	0	0	0
Dinner				
weight watchers bowtie pasta w/ cheese	13	40	8.5	295
ice cream	2	17	8	140
Opt Snack				
	48	116	22	866

30 elip
5|5|5 walk/ run

circuit (did really hard ready for 3x next week!

– salad

Date Tuesday 9/14/99	Protein	Carbs	Fats	Calories
Breakfast				
cereal w/ skim milk	14	36	0	190
Mid Morning				
Lunch				
peanut/jelly	9	29	16	330
2 cups milk	8	13	0	160
Mid afternoon				
sm. lasagna				
cup tomatoes cantelope apple				
piece angel food cake				
yogurt/wheat	7	19	0	115
Dinner				
lg salad (mush/onions)				
wrap (3 slices turkey)				
quarter pounder w/ fries				
Opt Snack				
water	114	168	48	1815
llll				

Wrap
180 cal
4 fat
7 pro
34 carb

Tabo
30 cal
1 fat
1 pro
3 carb

Hum
50 cal
2 fat
3 pro
5 carb

45 eliptical
circuit 2x
(increased to
18 reps)
100 jump rope

turkey
30 cal
1 carb
2 pro
0 fat

not including
mid-afternoon

Date Thurs 9/16/99	Protein	Carbs	Fats	Calories
Breakfast				
apple				
Mid Morning				
Lunch				
peanut butter jelly sandwich	9	29	1u	330
Mid afternoon				
5 graham crackers	5	59	4	270
Dinner				
chicken w/ bbq sauce				200
2 slices small pizza				
1 popsicle				
Opt Snack				

(no workout, depressed!)

Workout Log

This is the workout Debbie put me on when I was losing my weight.

Machine/Exercise	Date	Sets	Reps	Weight
Push-ups (tight Abs)		2-3	15-20	
squats & side leg lifts		2-3	15-20	10
over head tricep extensions		2-3	15-20	8-10
low squat → pliés				
one-arm rows		2-3	15-20	12-15
steps-up ē leg kick backs		2-3	15-20	12-15
upright rows		2-3	15-20	8
bicep curls (full/partial reps)		2-3	15-10-15	8
abdominals : ① Ab curl		2	10	8
② straight-leg lifts - straight scissors flutters		all 10	seconds	